D0912325

Medical Governance

Select Titles in the
American Governance and Public Policy Series

Series Editors: Gerard W. Boychuk, Karen Mossberger, and Mark C. Rom

Medical Governance

Values, Expertise, and Interests in Organ Transplantation

BAKER COLLEGE OF
CLINTON TWP. LIBRARY

David L. Weimer

Georgetown University Press
Washington, DC

© 2010 by Georgetown University Press. All rights reserved. No part of this book may be reproduced or utilized in any form or by any means, electronic or mechanical, including photocopying and recording, or by any information storage and retrieval system, without permission in writing from the publisher.

Library of Congress Cataloging-in-Publication Data

Weimer, David Leo.
  Medical governance : values, expertise, and interests in organ transplantation / David L. Weimer.
     p. ; cm.
  Includes bibliographical references and index.
  ISBN 978-1-58901-631-6 (pbk. : alk. paper)
  1. Organ Procurement and Transplantation Network (United States) 2. Procurement of organs, tissues, etc.—United States. 3. Transplantation of organs, tissues, etc.—United States. I. Title.
  [DNLM: 1. Organ Procurement and Transplantation Network (United States) 2. Organ Transplantation—legislation & jurisprudence—United States. 3. Government Regulation—United States. 4. Tissue and Organ Procurement—legislation & jurisprudence—United States.
  WO 690 W422m 2010]
  RD129.5.W45 2010
  617.9'54—dc22

                                                                          2009024524

∞ This book is printed on acid-free paper meeting the requirements of the American National Standard for Permanence in Paper for Printed Library Materials.

15 14 13 12 11 10   9 8 7 6 5 4 3 2
First printing

Printed in the United States of America

To Melanie, my heroine

Contents

Illustrations

Preface

My interest in organ transplantation began more than a decade ago with a driveway moment. I had tuned the car radio to *All Things Considered* on National Public Radio as I was about to leave a parking spot. A story about the controversy then under way over the allocation of cadaveric livers among U.S. transplant centers was just beginning. It caught my attention enough that I stayed put until it ended. I was most intrigued by the idea of organ allocation rules being determined by a private organization. It seemed puzzling that the federal government would delegate authority to make rules with immediate life and death consequences to a private organization.

Over the next few years I began learning about organ transplantation and its governance. The process was slow, largely because organ transplantation was usually my third or fourth research project. I made some progress when I obtained the extensive docket for the U.S. Department of Health and Human Services rulemaking that was the primary focus of the liver allocation controversy. It was not, however, until I moved to the University of Wisconsin–Madison, with its convenient proximity to the Hilton Hotel at O'Hare International Airport, where committees of the Organ Procurement and Transplantation Network (OPTN) met, that I gave organ transplantation serious attention and began realizing its broader implications for medical governance. Attending a number of these committee meetings as an observer made clear to me that the OPTN provides a framework for actually implementing evidence-based medicine, facilitating the combination of statistical evidence with the tacit knowledge of practitioners to develop rules that not only allocated extremely valuable resources but also promoted effective treatment. This led me to the central question addressed in this book: Is the OPTN, a private rulemaker, a useful model for effective governance in other medical contexts?

To answer this question I decided to look closely at OPTN decision processes, or, in case study terminology, to engage in inductive process tracing. I began by looking at liver allocation rules, which were at the heart of the controversy surrounding the OPTN during the late 1990s. I then turned to kidney allocation, in terms of both the slow evolution of rules to reduce racial disparity and more recent efforts to reformulate rules more fundamentally to place greater emphasis on maximizing the number of life-years provided by the limited supply of cadaveric organs. Realizing that allocation rules have implications for the supply of transplant organs from both deceased and live donors, I also considered policies relevant to organ supply. These cases, particularly those dealing with organ allocation, are the primary empirical basis of my assessment of the OPTN as a form of medical governance. They reflect the extensive use of documents, supplementary interviews with participants, and direct observation of committee meetings.

As a social scientist, I face the problems of making inferences about, and generalizations from, a single case. How do I know that the outcomes I observe differ from those that would have occurred under other governance arrangements? Would similar decision patterns occur if the governance arrangement were replicated in other contexts?

My answer to the internal validity question rests primarily on the assertion that prior research tells us a lot about the outcomes we can expect from traditional agency regulation, the most likely alternative to the OPTN. Although less than epistemologically ideal, I attribute differences between outcomes I observe and those I would expect under the regulatory counterfactual to the OPTN. My confidence is bolstered at least somewhat by my earlier work reviewing other cases of private rulemaking, from the allocation of agricultural production quotas to the assignment of Internet domain names. These cases showed the functional advantage of technical efficiency, though not necessarily in promoting social welfare, and the political advantage of blame avoidance for government officials.

Answering the external validity question is more difficult. As a social scientist, it would not be unreasonable to give it little attention—understanding how the OPTN operates is itself worthwhile, especially in view of the importance of what it does. However, as a policy analyst, I see the payoff of the research primarily in terms of its contribution to the better design of governance. Medical governance has received relatively little scholarly attention, especially in terms of the sorts of arrangements that can promote evidence-based medicine. Understanding the circumstances in which private rulemaking is likely to be feasible and desirable contributes to more informed choices of governance arrangements. In addition to making arguments about the important features of the OPTN and how they contribute to observed outcomes, I offer two possible applications of private rulemaking. Using it to achieve interoperable electronic records involves only an incremental change from the governance arrangements already being put in place. Using it to promote evidence-based surgery is a more fundamental innovation.

I hope that readers find my account of the OPTN interesting and my assertions about the potential for private rulemaking persuasive. I also hope they find my arguments about the importance of studying medical governance convincing. I will be delighted if other researchers agree and contribute in-depth studies of other institutional forms to the enterprise. In complex situations we should expect new governance arrangements to be rarely created de novo, but rather based on replications of familiar designs or assembled from common features. One of our important, but too often neglected, tasks as policy researchers is to expand understanding of the advantages and disadvantages of those designs.

Acknowledgments

In a number of places in this book I use data from the Scientific Registry of Transplant Patients through the Organ Procurement and Transplantation Network, calling for the following acknowledgment and disclaimer: "This work was supported in part by Health Resources and Services Administration contract 231–00–0115. The content is the responsibility of the authors alone and does not necessarily reflect the views or policies of the Department of Health and Human Services, nor does mention of trade names, commercial products, or organizations imply endorsement by the U.S. Government." It also draws on work I have previously published. Parts of chapter 1 originally appeared in "Medical Governance: Are We Ready to Prescribe?" *Journal of Policy Analysis and Management* 26, no. 2 (2007): 217–39; parts of chapter 2 originally appeared in "The Puzzle of Private Rulemaking: Scientific Expertise, Flexibility, and Blame Avoidance in Regulation," *Public Administration Review* 66, no. 4 (2006): 569–82; and much of chapter 5 originally appeared in "Public and Private Regulation of Organ Transplantation: Liver Allocation and the Final Rule," *Journal of Health Politics, Policy and Law* 32, no. 1 (2007): 9–49.

I am grateful to the Robert M. La Follette School of Public Affairs at the University of Wisconsin–Madison, which on several occasions provided financial support for summer salary and project assistants.

Many people helped me at various stages of this research. I apologize in advance to those I fail to identify by name—the extended period over which I conducted my research makes it difficult for me to recall everyone who provided assistance or advice. Many participants in OPTN committees, both transplant professionals and patient representatives, have my thanks for taking time to talk with me at meetings. I would particularly like to thank Richard B. Freeman, who was very generous in offering comments on my analysis of the Final Rule controversy. Several staff members of the United Network for Organ Sharing facilitated my efforts to gather information: Ciara Samana, Deanna Parker, Karl J. McCleary, Lorraine Sitler, and especially Doug Heiney, who assisted me throughout the project. Richard Durbin of the Division of Transplantation, U.S. Department of Health and Human Services was very helpful at the early stage of the project. I thank the students who served as project assistants, especially Laura Flamand-Gomez, Katie Croake, Stephanie Caucutt, Dan Walters, and David Stepien. Many others have offered advice or assistance along the way, including Eugene Bardach, Ivar Bleiklie, David Canon, Menzie Chinn, Erik Devereux, Stan Engerman, Edward Friedman, William T. Gormley Jr., Eric Hanushek, Robert Haveman, Carolyn Heinrich, Pamela Herd, Karen Holden, Hank Jenkins-Smith, Stéphane Lavertu, Laurence Lynn Jr., Melanie Manion, Ted Marmor, John Mendeloff, Donald Moynihan, Dana Mukamel, Gregory Nemet, Thomas Oliver, Eric Patashnik, Christine Rothmayer, Mark Schlesinger, Julie Schneider, Louise Trubek, Dan Walters, Joseph White, Susan Yackee, Aidan Vining, Jonathan Zeitlin, and two anonymous reviewers. I also thank Gail Grella and Don Jacobs of Georgetown University Press for their encouragement. In addition, I thank participants in the Workshop on Politics of Biomedicine at the 2002 European Consortium for Political Research, the Public Policy Seminar at Simon Fraser University, and the La Follette School of Public Affairs Seminar Series. Of course, I alone bear responsibility for any errors and all the opinions expressed in this book.

Abbreviations and Acronyms

ACIP	Advisory Committee on Immunization Practices
AHIC	American Health Information Community
CDC	Centers for Disease Control and Prevention
CHBRP	California Health Benefits Review Program
CMS	Centers for Medicare and Medicaid Services
CPRA	calculated panel reactive antibody
CREG	cross-reactive antigen group
DPI	donor profile index
DRG	diagnostic related group
DSA	donation service area
DT	dialysis time (years on dialysis)
ECD	expanded criteria donors
EPA	Environmental Protection Agency
ESRD	end-stage renal disease
FDA	Food and Drug Administration
HEDIS	Health Plan and Employers Data Information Set
HHS	Department of Health and Human Services
HLA	human leucocyte antigen
HRSA	Health Resources and Services Administration
IOM	Institute of Medicine
JCAHO	Joint Commission on Accreditation of Healthcare Organizations
KARS	Kidney Allocation Review Subcommittee
KAS	kidney allocation score
KPSAM	kidney-pancreas simulated allocation model
KPTC	Kidney and Pancreas Transplantation Committee
KTC	Kidney Transplantation Committee
LAS	lung allocation score
LYFT	life-years from transplant
MEDCAC	Medicare Evidence Development & Coverage Advisory Committee
MedPAC	Medicare Payment Advisory Commission

MedSAVE	Medicare Surgery Assessment Volunteers for Effectiveness
MELD	model for end-stage liver disease
MOTTEP	National Minority Organ/Tissue Transplant Education Program
MPSC	Membership and Professional Standards Committee
NAMER	National Archive for Medical Electronic Records
NAO	network administrative organization
NICE	National Institute for Health and Clinical Excellence
OPO	organ procurement organization
OPTN	Organ Procurement and Transplantation Network
PELD	pediatric end-stage liver disease
PRA	panel reactive antibody
RRB	regional review boards
SEOPP	South-Eastern Regional Organ Procurement Program
SGR	sustainable growth rate
SRTR	Scientific Registry of Transplant Recipients
TOTC	Thoracic Organ Transplantation Committee
UKAM^{SM}	UNOS Kidney Allocation Model
UNOS	United Network for Organ Sharing
UPMC	University of Pittsburgh Medical Center

1

Medical Governance
Important but Neglected

Governments throughout the industrialized world make decisions that fundamentally affect the quality and accessibility of medical care. In the United States, despite the absence of universal health insurance, these decisions have great influence on the practice of medicine, and, because of the absence of universal health insurance, occur in a great variety of institutional contexts. We see direct federal provision of medical care through the Veterans Administration, federal funding and regulation through Medicare, federal and state funding and regulation through Medicaid, federal funding of health services research, and state regulation of private group health insurance and entry into the health-related professions, to name the most familiar. Each of these contexts has a particular form of governance, which, following Laurence Lynn, Carolyn Heinrich, and Carolyn Hill, consists of the "regimes of laws, administrative rules, judicial rulings, and practices that constrain, prescribe, and enable government activity," broadly defined (2000, 3). One less familiar form is private rulemaking, an arrangement in which stakeholders exercise explicitly delegated authority over the development and adoption of rules within the framework of a nongovernmental organization, or in the terminology of network theory, a network administrative organization. The Organ Procurement and Transplantation Network (OPTN) is an example: organ allocation policies with life and death consequences are determined by representatives of transplant centers and other stakeholders. How effectively does this delegation integrate expertise and values to produce fair and efficient rules? The answer is important—for organ transplantation policy, obviously, but more generally for assessing the advantages and disadvantages of private rulemaking compared to other forms of medical governance.

The opportunities for improving health through better governance are obvious to even the casual reader of the newspaper. For example, an Institute of Medicine study reports that as many as ninety-eight thousand Americans die prematurely each year because of medical errors (Kohn, Corrigan, and Donaldson 2000, 1). More recently, another Institute of Medicine study indicates—amazingly—that on average each hospital patient in the United States is subject to one medication error per day (Aspden et al. 2007). These medication errors lead to approximately 1.5 million injuries and inflict $3.5 billion in costs each year. Better medical governance could help reduce the frequency and cost of such errors by establishing realistic standards, promoting compliance through changes in professional norms or regulations, or advocating changes in relevant framework laws.

A few preliminary comments on medical governance are appropriate. Most important, medical governance should not be viewed in terms of a single institution, but rather as the collection of the particular institutional arrangements for governance that appear throughout a complex health care system. The nature of health care and our goals for the heath care system, however, make it useful to view these institutions within the broad category of medical governance. Against a backdrop of changing knowledge about the possibility, efficacy, and safety of medical treatments, a large informational asymmetry between patients and providers typically complicates market exchange. Because of the potential for medical care to improve health and to prolong life, many see fair access to it as important for a good society. Medical care is also expensive and thus access has implications for the availability of other things people value.

These particular characteristics of medical care raise the importance of what we generally seek to achieve in all governance: technical efficiency, democratic accountability, and promotion of social values, including economy. Technical efficiency entails allowing rapidly changing medical expertise, based on both scientific evidence and tacit knowledge, to be continuously integrated into decision-making processes. Democratic accountability involves both maintaining appropriate oversight by elected officials and promoting authentic public participation in decision making. It also entails balancing a variety of values, including equity and compassion, that may at times conflict with other goals. The challenge of promoting social values involves finding arrangements that facilitate the consideration of costs and benefits, broadly defined in decision making. Medical governance deserves our attention because of the importance, and difficulty, of finding balanced responses to these challenges.

Looking Ahead: Four Likely Sources of Demand for Advice about Medical Governance

John Kingdon argues that major policy changes occur when there is a confluence of the "problem stream," the "policy stream," and the "political stream" (1984). That is, some events focus political attention on a problem for which a policy community, those in the public, private, and not-for-profit sectors concerned with the issue, can offer a solution. Unfortunately, this framework, and related ones like "punctuated equilibrium" that have followed, do not tell us when such opportunities are likely to materialize or how one might go about creating them. Nonetheless, these studies make a strong empirical case that instances of nonincremental change do occur (Jones and Baumgartner 2005). Because opportunities are transitory, it is unlikely that researchers working in the policy stream will be able to offer any advice about governance based on research not already completed or at least well under way. If researchers are not ready with well-thought-out solutions, then the opportunity will be lost or exploited using whatever ideas that happen to be at hand. Knowing more about the advantages and disadvantages of alternative forms of medical governance increases the likelihood that viable policy alternatives will be available when policy windows open.

One can imagine at least four sorts of opportunities arising that would call for researchers to offer advice about medical governance.

First, and the longest odds, a demand may arise in the context of serious consideration of universal health insurance. This might be prompted by concern among businesses about their growing employee health insurance costs and the implications of these costs for global competitiveness. It might follow a political landslide, as did the adoption of Medicare. Because no society can be rich enough to cover every possible medical procedure for every person, some mechanisms would have to be included to delineate what was and was not covered. For example, imagine a system that emphasized reducing catastrophic risk but also sought to promote preventive care. What medical interventions would be considered too risky or too costly? What routine diagnostic tests would be considered essential components of preventive care? The governance arrangements put in place to answer these questions would largely determine the impact of universal health insurance on the medical care actually delivered and the health outcomes this care produces.

Yet even informed discussions of universal health insurance rarely delve very deeply into issues of governance. Consider the last major push for universal coverage in the United States, the Clinton health plan. Jacob Hacker notes that, compared to the attention paid to financing and cost control, "the administrative architecture of the plan received scant attention" with few advisors asking if the proposed institutions "could actually be created or expected to operate effectively" (1997, 127). Is the policy research community any better prepared to address questions of governance now than it was in 1993?

Second, within the current framework of the government as a major provider of medical care for veterans and the copurchaser of medical care for the elderly and the poor, demands may arise to put evidence-based medicine into practice as called for by many prominent health policy experts (e.g., Dranove 2003; Cutler 2004; Neumann 2005). A small army of physicians, epidemiologists, economists, and other social scientists funded by the National Institutes of Health, private foundations, and pharmaceutical companies is already seeking empirical evidence about the effectiveness of various sorts of medical care. A small amount of this work even assesses some elements of the governance of health care delivery, such as the difference between the delivery of services by for-profit versus nonprofit organizations (Forbes, Hill, and Lynn 2006). Although it is not clear whether there is enough or the right kind of such research, what is clear is the absence of institutional arrangements for effectively moving such evidence into medical practice—the gap between the discovery of more efficacious treatments and their incorporation into routine patient care in the United States is currently about fifteen to twenty years (IOM 2001, 145).

As an illustration of the current problem of bringing evidence into practice, and therefore the substantive opportunity it offers, consider the case of arthroscopy of the knee presented by Alan Gerber and Erik Patashnik (2006). Unlike pharmaceuticals, which undergo extensive clinical trials before being marketed in the United States, surgical procedures typically come into use based on the accounts surgeons provide of their impacts on a series of patients. There have, however, been a few random-assignment surgery studies in which patients in the control group received an incision so that neither they nor the physicians assessing effects after surgery could tell whether they had the procedure. The most prominent of these sham surgery studies, published in the *New England Journal of Medicine* (Moseley et al. 2002), assessed arthroscopy, a common treatment for osteoarthritis of the knee. Over a two-year follow-up, the study of 180 patients found no statistical difference in terms of pain or function between the treatment and control groups. Because at least one hundred thousand such surgeries are performed every year in the United States at as much as five thousand dollars per surgery, the potential resource implications of this finding are large. The Centers for Medicare and Medicaid Services considered the study and even removed one type of the surgery from automatic coverage under Medicare, although local Medicare contractors could, and still do, generally cover it. Thus, in the face of actual opposition from orthopedists and potential opposition from other specialists, the finding has had little if any immediate impact. One can imagine alternative governance arrangements that would increase the chances that Medicare reimbursements would more closely reflect available evidence about effectiveness.

Agencies attempting to apply evidence-based medicine even risk attack if they challenge the efficacy of lucrative procedures. A prominent example is the response elicited by a review of available literature on spinal fusion by the Agency for Health Care Policy and Research, the forerunner of the currently operating Agency for Healthcare Research and Quality. Its multidisciplinary team reviewed the available literature and concluded that there were few scientifically supported indications for spinal fusion and recommended nonsurgical treatments for most of the conditions for which it was being used (Deyo et al. 1997). In response, in 1995 the North American Spine Society started a nearly successful letter writing campaign to get Congress to eliminate funds for the agency (Gray, Gusmano, and Collins 2003). Although it survived, the agency stopped producing the sort of practice reviews that prompted the attack. Evidence-based medicine requires robust governance arrangements to both produce good assessments and translate them into practice.

Third, proposals for fundamental change in the nature of the health care system, which require major accompanying changes in governance arrangements, may gain traction among the public and stakeholders in the medical system. Consider, for example, the call by Michael Porter and Elizabeth Olmsted Teisberg for value-based competition (2006). On the one hand, they optimistically see the movement toward value-based competition as coming primarily from within the health care system: "Fortunately, government is not the key to health care reform. We believe that health care reform can come, and will come, largely from within" (326). On the other hand, they recognize that government can play a number of important roles, such as initiating a "systemwide government information strategy" (343) to mandate the collection of results information. They only briefly suggest a number of possible governance arrangements for implementing the strategy. Interestingly, they point to the OPTN, which has overseen the development of a data base that longitudinally follows all transplant recipients in the United States, as a possible model. However, they identify neither the essential elements of the governance arrangements they list, nor their relative advantages and disadvantages. The choice among these arrangements would certainly affect the nature of the information strategy adopted and the effectiveness of its implementation. Informing this choice seems essential for increasing the chances of achieving their desired reform. More generally, any major reform will pose similar demands for advice about comparative forms of governance.

Fourth, and most likely, a demand for advice about medical governance may arise from the fiscal pressure put on the federal government by Medicare and on state and federal governments by Medicaid (Rivlin and Antos 2007). Many observers see explicit rationing of services in terms of their cost-effectiveness as an inevitable consequence of rising medical costs. Indeed, to some extent this is actually being done by the Oregon Health Services Commission. Henry Aaron, William Schwartz, and Melissa Cox argue that "continued growth of health care expenditures will therefore force Americans to consider heretofore unthinkable ways to limit spending" (2005, 147). If they are right, shouldn't health policy researchers be preparing to offer advice about how this can and should be done?

Governance: The Gap between Research and Prescription

Recognizing the importance of governance arrangements to the implementation and management, and therefore to the outcomes, of public policies, a number of scholars have sought in recent years to focus research attention directly on governance (Lynn, Heinrich, and Hill 2001; Meier and O'Toole 2006). A few have even focused attention specifically on medical governance (Trubek et al. 2008). Yet, one might ask, why is it necessary to adopt a new perspective on a topic that one would expect to be a central concern of economics, political science, public administration, and law? A brief review of the most relevant research streams in these disciplines provides an answer.

Economics

Consider economics first. Two related but distinct theoretical approaches, agency theory and transaction cost theory, provide frameworks for most of the economic research dealing with governance. Each framework focuses on the design of efficient contracts.

Agency theory in its broadest conception sees firms and other organizations as the nexus of contracts among owners, workers, suppliers, and customers (Jensen and Meckling 1976). Following work on syndicates (Wilson 1968) and insurance and information (Spence and Zeckhauser 1971), Steven Ross (1973) introduced a formal framework, the principal-agent model, for analyzing contracting in situations in which an agent enjoys an informational advantage relative to a principal seeking some action by the agent. The theory has evolved to consider various types of agent actions and information that are hidden, or imperfectly observed, by the principal as well as the implications of multiple principals, multiple tasks, and adverse selection among multiple agents. Most elaborations of the theory have been developed within the context of very stylized and relatively simple institutional arrangements (for accessible reviews of the formal literature, see Holmstrom and Tirole 1989; Sappington 1991; Banks 1995). The testable implications of the theory have been explored in many contexts, especially with respect to wage contracts and executive compensation. Although some studies appear to verify predictions of the theory with respect to contract design, the overall evidence is "hardly overwhelming" (Prendergast 1999, 21).

The inherent difficulty of measuring contributions of individual agents' output to many publicly provided goods and services, as well as the constraints on bureaucratic principals imposed by civil service rules to prevent the diversion of public resources to partisan purposes, limit the opportunities for the substitution of incentives for monitoring, the central thrust of principal-agent theory. Even when output can be measured, bureaucratic principals may forgo efficient incentive contracts they consider too costly in terms of their personal interests (Miller and Whitford 2006). Consequently, aside from the general admonition to "get the incentives right," the formal principal-agent literature offers relatively little advice directly relevant to the design of governance mechanisms in complex situations.

The related, but less formal, transaction cost theory emphasizes the problem of contract compliance. The transaction cost approach was introduced by Ronald Coase (1937, 1960) and prominently applied to governance by Oliver Williamson (1985). Most commonly, transaction costs are defined as "the resources used to establish and maintain property rights" (Allen 1991, 1). These costs depend on uncertainty about future contingencies and the actions of those participating in the transaction (Slater and Spencer 2000). Although transaction cost theory has been used to analyze a wide variety of organizational forms (Shelanski and Klein 1995; Macher and Richman 2008), it has probably had its greatest impact in informing the choice between producing goods and services within organizations or contracting for them with other organizations.

The transaction cost approach considers bargaining and opportunism costs as well as production costs in assessing alternative institutional arrangements (Globerman and Vining 1996; Vining and Globerman 1998). Production costs are simply the opportunity costs in terms of the real resources required to produce a good or service. Bargaining costs include resources expended in finding potential contracting partners, assessing their likely performance, writing detailed and mutually agreeable contracts, addressing unforeseen circumstances that arise during contract execution, monitoring contract compliance, and resolving any disputes arising over contract compliance. Opportunism costs are the losses one party to the contract suffers when another party acts in bad faith to manipulate the agreed terms. Bargaining and opportunism costs generally depend on the complexity of the production task, the number of potential contractors who can contest for the contract, and the extent to which the production process uses assets that, once created, have much lower value in alternative uses. The design problem is to choose institutional arrangements to minimize the sum of production, bargaining, and opportunism costs.

Empirical work has addressed the implication of the theory for the relative efficiency of organizational forms (Vining and Boardman 1992; Dilger, Moffitt, and Struyk 1997; Hodge 2000). It has also investigated specific implications of the theory, such as the relationships between investments in monitoring and the risk of opportunism (Brown and Potoski 2003) and asset specificity and contracting out for services (Lyons 1995).

Agency and transaction cost theories offer insights about the uses of incentives and monitoring in governance arrangements. They generally do not provide the basis for the wholesale design of new institutions. One prominent exception was the simultaneous ascending auction of radio spectrum developed for the Federal Communication Commission in the mid-1990s. Economic theory guided its basic design. Although auctions are relatively simple institutions compared to a complex bureaucracy with multiple goals and tasks, this one was especially complex because it involved simultaneous bidding on many geographic-spectrum combinations. The designers appropriately went beyond economic theory. To create a well-functioning institution in light of the problems previously encountered in other countries with ascending auctions and those suggested through extensive simulations, more than 130 pages of regulations were required (McAfee and McMillian 1996). One can think of these pages as a measure of the gap between simple theory and practical prescription.

Political Science

Research in political science often considers questions potentially relevant to the design of public governance arrangements. The scope of these projects has ranged from the cross-national comparison of political regimes (Powell 2000; Cheibub and Limongi 2002) to the impact of specific governance mechanisms such as negotiated rulemaking (Langbein and Kerwin 2000) and consensual rulemaking more generally (Balla and Wright 2003), private and public standard setting (Cheit 1990), the representation of consumer interests before public utility commissions (Gormley 1983), mechanisms for deliberative democracy (Goodin and Dryzek 2006), and public participation in Medicaid reform (Grogan and Gusmano 2005). One aspect of governance, the legislative control of the bureaucracy, has been the dominant concern within the discipline in recent years, however.

Recognizing the difficulty Congress faces in carrying out oversight (McCubbins and Schwartz 1984), Matthew McCubbins, Roger Noll, and Barry Weingast argue that the legislative coalition that creates a bureau can control its discretion by imposing various administrative procedures at its inception (1987, 1989). These procedures, which may require the production and revelation of various sorts of information to make actions more visible to legislators or interest groups, facilitate oversight by reducing the informational asymmetry between the coalition (principal) and the bureau (agent). The coalition may also stack the deck in favor of its preferences by enfranchising particular interest groups in the bureau's decision making processes, for example, by specifying the composition of advisory committees (Balla and Wright 2001). Within this general framework, the delegation and control of bureaucratic discretion by legislatures has received considerable empirical attention, both within the United States (Epstein and O'Halloran 1999) and comparatively (Huber and Shipan 2002).

The focus on the control of discretion, however, is almost certainly too narrow to serve as the basis for effective prescription for several reasons. First, as Jonathan Bendor and Adam Meirowitz note, relaxing some of the common assumptions of the model move the results closer to more traditional views of hierarchical organization as yielding superior outcomes through delegation to specialists and experts (2004). Also, with few exceptions (Fiorina 1982), the models do not recognize situations in which strong control is politically undesirable because the risks of blame for unfavorable outcomes are not offset enough by the opportunities for credit claiming (Weimer 2006). Controlling discretion is surely important, but bureaus usually receive delegations of authority because they can gather, process, or act on information more effectively and with less political risk than the legislature can. A framework broad enough to support prescription should consider the advantages and disadvantages of alternative ways of achieving the desired benefits of delegated discretion as well as the ways of controlling it.

Second, as Kenneth Meier and Laurence O'Toole note, the implementation of modern public policy typically involves more than one bureau (2006). Their analysis of legislation passed by the 103rd Congress, for example, found that only 10 percent of laws specified implementation through a single agency (56). They further argued that increasingly implementation takes place through complex networks that do not fit the control frameworks political scientists generally use—agents and principals are multiple and not necessarily situated in neat hierarchical relationships. Individual models have selectively incorporated many of these complications, but still fall short of capturing much of the complexity of the contexts in which delegation decisions must be made.

Third, as Meier and O'Toole also note, the control perspective largely ignores the role of the values held by bureaucrats (2006). The appropriate set of values for unelected public officials has been one of the central concerns of public administration scholars. For example, John Rohr argues that public officials have a responsibility to inform their actions with an understanding of the constitutional underpinnings of their duties (1980). More recently, Anthony Bertelli and Laurence Lynn consider bureaucracy from the perspective of the separation of powers to develop a precept of managerial responsibility based on judgment, balance, rationality, and accountability (2006). The key ideas are that bureaucratic performance can be affected by the inculcation of specific norms within administrators and that the personnel system can be used to select and advance administrators adhering to these norms.

Whereas political science offers surprisingly little on the nitty-gritty of governance design, it does offer an abundance of theory and empirical research relevant to understanding policy processes. For example, path dependence recognizes that policy choices at one time often affect the costs and benefits borne by relevant interests that would result from policy changes in the future (Pierson 2000; Page 2006). Consequently, initial choices, including those adopted for seemingly random reasons, can make future changes more or less politically difficult. For instance, the desire of firms to provide an allowable benefit to workers under the wage controls of World War II spurred the growth of a private health insurance industry that subsequently helped block national health insurance and contributed to the choice of using private intermediaries to administer Medicare. At a more micro level, policies and routines adopted when institutions of governance were established often have substantial influence on the way the institutions respond to changing circumstances in their environments.

Public Administration

Public administration scholars have been criticized for not being specific enough about defining and inculcating desirable norms (Meier and O'Toole 2006). The task is particularly challenging in the context of the governance of science and medicine, where managerial responsibility must either incorporate or be exercised in conjunction with professional norms, where, following Eliot Freidson, a profession is "an occupation which has assumed a dominant position in a division of labor, so that it gains control over the determination of the substance of its own work" (1970, xvii). In science, epistemological values underpin professional norms—awareness of how the community of scholars comes to know something is central. In medicine, similar values are important, but responsibility for the well-being of the patient dominates.

Efforts to create effective governance of science and medicine should accommodate these professional norms. Along the lines Eugene Bardach and Robert Kagan suggest in the context of the regulatory inspectorate (1982), norms are sometimes resources to tap in designing governance arrangements. When strong, they may counter or reshape narrow self-interest in desirable ways, perhaps making it easier to maintain a common mission among those directly involved in the governance arrangements. They may also change the extent and nature of desirable oversight by elected representatives. For example, it may be more appropriate to rely on physicians to speak for patient interests than health insurance firms. In some situations, it may be possible to assign tasks to groups with strong norms, either professional or social, that reinforce material incentives. For instance, casinos in British Columbia are monitored by members of charitable organizations that receive a portion of the province's share of revenue (Vining and Weimer 1997).

Strong professional norms may facilitate, or even demand, greater delegation of authority. Alice Rivlin, the first director of the Congressional Budget Office, offered the following advice in a commencement address at the Rand Graduate School: "The best rule for politicians for dealing with generals, admirals, and doctors may be this: put the money on the stump and run" (1983, 6). Her admonition recognizes the difficulty politicians face in dealing with communities with strong professional identities and norms. It also recognizes that the professional norms, if strong enough, may enable politicians to rely on the professionals to behave in predictable ways. The problem of governance then becomes one of creating situations that align norm-induced behavior with public policy goals.

Such alignment, however, may be complicated when members of the organization come from professions with conflicting norms. For example, the procedural norms of lawyers may conflict with those for promoting substantive values, such as welfare of the patient, protection of endangered species, or actuarial integrity. The institutional design problem then becomes selectively favoring professional expertise in decision-making processes in which the particular norms of the profession support good policy decisions and retard bad ones.

Moving beyond the traditional focus on processes within agencies, public administration scholars have in recent years begun to address the organizational complexity generally encountered in the implementation and management of public policy through the study of interorganizational networks, that is, "groups of three or more legally autonomous organizations that work together to achieve not only their own goals but also a collective goal" (Provan and Kenis 2008, 3). A small but growing number of studies consider the collection of organizations making up a network rather than focus on a specific organization within a network (Morrissey, Tausig, and Lindsey 1985; Provan, Fish, and Sydow 2007). In an influential study within public administration, Keith Proven and H. Brinton Milward assess the performance of mental health networks in four locations (1995). They inductively develop a number of propositions about the implications of network structure and environment on performance. Specifically, they propose that networks coordinated and integrated centrally through a single core agency are likely to be more effective than even cohesive networks with decentralized integration.

Nonetheless, the consequences of the alternative forms of governance of networks remain relatively understudied (Provan, Fish, and Sydow 2007; Provan and Kenis 2008).

The possibilities range from voluntary participation in coordination efforts by members of the network to an administrative entity, a network administrative organization (NAO), specifically established to govern the network. Provan and Patrick Kenis propose that NAOs are likely to be the most effective form of governance for achieving desired network-level outcomes "when trust is moderately to widely shared among network participants…, when there are a moderate number to many network participants, when network-level goal consensus is moderately high, and when need for network-level competencies are high" (2008, 13). They see NAOs as providing balance between efficient operation and inclusive decision making as well as between internal and external legitimacy.

Perhaps the most prescriptive body of social science research on governance deals with the varieties of response to a generic problem of natural resource management, the preservation of common pool resources. Over the course of her career, Elinor Ostrom has studied numerous self-governance arrangements that have enabled those sharing natural resources to avoid extreme depletion without resort to either privatization or external regulation (1990). A number of design principles emerge from her comparative research. For example, graduated sanctions on those who violate appropriation rules appear to contribute to the preservation of common pool resources. So does the availability of local arenas for resolving conflict among appropriators at low cost. One can imagine a group facing a new common pool resource problem applying these principles to develop a governance arrangement that increased the chances of avoiding the rapid depletion of the resource predicted by economic theory.

Law

Governance has always been a central concern of public law scholars, though often with a narrow focus on the operation of existing institutions within the framework of legal theory. Some of this work explicitly develops the trade-offs among alternative forms. For example, Jody Freeman does so in the context of thinking about governance as generally involving negotiation among private and public actors during the design, implementation, and enforcement of rules (2000). As such, she challenges the notion of hierarchical accountability and argued for a research agenda that focuses explicitly on the relationships between public and private actors and their shared responsibility. Other examples include assessments of management-based regulation (Coglianese and Lazer 2003) and information forcing regulation (Karkkainen 2006).

Drawing more heavily on the empirical social sciences, especially sociology, law and society scholars have sought to expand thinking about the range and functions of the institutions of governance. The claimed evolution beginning with repressive law to achieve order, then autonomous law to tame repression, and eventually responsive law to achieve substantive goals (Nonet and Selznik 1978) leads to contemporary concerns about how legal institutions actually affect society. Louise Trubek and her colleagues refer specifically to medical governance in arguing that "new institutions that advance good quality medical care should be able to include both the traditional knowledge of the good practitioner and the other knowledge that comes from the patient, community ethics, statistical analysis, and comparative practice" (2008, 7). Understanding the extent to which institutions actually incorporate these sorts of knowledge and values requires detailed empirical investigation as well as theory.

Confronting Complexity

The research projects in economics, political science, public administration, and law all offer insights to help design and choose among governance arrangements. Where it is possible to study multiple units, such as local government contracts, major pieces of legislation, or common pool resources, theories can be tested or inductively developed. In U.S. health policy, this is often done taking advantage of variations across states, and is likely to be especially important as a number of states move to provide universal health insurance for their residents. Researchers have also sought to make international comparisons, though such studies are difficult to execute (Riker and Weimer 1995). Nonetheless, several such efforts in the medical area are exemplary. At one extreme, a specific substantive focus, such as policies governing assisted reproductive technologies, can facilitate comparison across a large number of countries (Bleiklie, Goggin, and Rothmayr 2004). Broader comparisons are also possible, though much more difficult to do well. For example, Carolyn Hughes Tuohy provided exceptionally rich accounts of the general evolution of medical governance in the United States, Britain, and Canada (1999). Obviously, comparisons of institutions cross-nationally suffer because it is not possible to hold constant differences in political institutions and national cultures. As Ted Marmor, Richard Freeman, and Kieke Okma discuss with insight, drawing valid policy lessons from even the best international comparisons is difficult (2005).

Whereas scholars seek to discover general truths about the world (and less nobly claim priority of discovery), politicians and policy designers seek to solve specific problems (and less nobly claim credit for solutions). When the political opportunity for solving a problem arises, it must be seized quickly or it will be lost as it is inevitably eclipsed by new problems or opportunities. Consequently, the pressures of acting expeditiously rarely allow for the design of governance arrangements from first principles. Rather, the more expedient course is to borrow from among the approaches already in use. Does an agency exist that already deals with a similar problem? If yes, then perhaps delegate the new authority to it. Is a network already dealing with the problem to some extent? If yes, then perhaps formalize its authority. Does the private sector provide a similar service to the one needed for the solution? If yes, then perhaps create incentives or introduce regulations of the private providers to implement the solution. Finding a governance arrangement already in operation has a number of advantages. Most important, it suggests the many details needed to create a workable governance arrangement in a complex world of existing and often overlapping organizational responsibilities, legal and constitutional constraints, demands for participation by stakeholders, and substantive requirements such as appropriate expertise and rapidity of action. Arrangements already in operation may also be more politically acceptable and present less risk of a major failure during implementation.

Governance scholarship can inform expedient choice by identifying the advantages and disadvantages of working models, as well as the prerequisites for realizing the advantages and the conditions contributing to the disadvantages that may be relevant to transfer of the model to other contexts. These tasks require a close look at the working models, including at least some of the outcomes they produce. Identifying the relevant prerequisites and conditions requires that the close look be more than just a description. It should take advantage of the general knowledge about governance that has accumulated to help focus on the most essential features of the working model. Where possible, it should contrast the working model with other forms of governance that would be likely alternatives.

I demonstrate this approach by analyzing the governance of organ transplantation in the United States. Organ transplantation is important in its own right. In mid-2008, the waiting list in the United States for solid organ transplants (kidneys, livers, hearts, lungs, pancreases, and intestines) had more than one hundred thousand registrants, more than quadruple the approximately twenty-four thousand patients waiting in 1990, and during 2008 more than seven thousand people died while waiting for organs (OPTN 2009). The persistent shortage of cadaveric organs has led to substantial increases in the numbers of kidneys and livers transplanted from live donors, raising issues of donor risk, especially with respect to livers. Transplants also involve substantial expenditures of health care resources. In 2008, the average billed charges in the United States for the 20 days before the transplant operation and the 180 days after ranged from $259,000 for kidneys to $1,121,800 for intestines (Hauboldt and Hanson 2008, 5). The availability and allocation of organs for transplant are certainly important public policy issues with literal life and death implications.

Organ transplantation also presents a particularly interesting and potentially important model of governance. Before 1984 the collection and allocation of cadaveric organs was governed largely through voluntary participation by organ transplant centers in a network with a self-governing NAO. In 1984 Congress statutorily created a strong NAO that provides a governance arrangement in which transplant centers and other stakeholders set the de facto rules for allocating scarce organs. The legislation also created a comprehensive data collection system that facilitates the sort of evidence-based research many observers see as necessary for improving the practice of medicine. The governance of organ transplantation thus combines the tacit knowledge of the stakeholders with strong scientific evidence.

The governance of organ transplantation raises a concern and poses a related puzzle. The concern is whether the participating stakeholders adequately represent society and appropriately weigh all the relevant values. The puzzle is why Congress would delegate the responsibility for making rules with life and death implications to a network of stakeholders. This question can be answered a number of ways. First, Congress realized that good rulemaking would require cutting-edge expertise that could be effectively provided only by the stakeholders. Second, Congress viewed direct involvement in organ allocation as having unfavorable prospects in terms of blame avoidance and credit claiming and therefore sought to remove the issue from the politics that would occur with agency rulemaking. Third, Congress saw the new governance arrangements as building on existing network cooperation; in other words, it was a design readily at hand. Investigating the validity of the premise underlying the first explanation is one of the major tasks of this book. The other explanations also are relevant to understanding what features of governance systems are likely to make them attractive to policymakers.

Roadmap

The remaining chapters of this book explore more fully the problem of medical governance, specifically, the extent to which the organ transplantation system provides a viable and desirable model of medical governance. Chapter 2 sets the stage by considering the trade-offs among values, expertise, and interests inherent in any system of governance. The trade-offs are framed initially by considering two extreme modes of governance: largely unregulated markets and traditional bureaucracy. These forms are the caricatures of opposing ideologies in the debate over expanding health insurance. Because neither is a viable form of governance for medicine, chapter 2 goes on to consider some of the important hybrid forms that are actually used. These include, first, varying reliance on advisory committees to help bureaus maintain adequate expertise in the face of rapidly evolving scientific and medical knowledge and, second, delegation of agenda setting authority by legislatures to advisory committees. The U.S. Food and Drug Administration's use of advisory committees in the drug and medical device approval process is an example of the former; the Oregon Health Plan is a prominent example of the latter. More generally, chapter 2 sets out private rulemaking as an alternative to public rulemaking for structuring medical governance.

The next five chapters focus explicitly on the governance of organ transplantation through private rulemaking. Chapter 3 provides a brief history of the OPTN and an overview of its structure and operations as an network administrative organization. Chapter 4 considers the governance of organ supply, including efforts to expand the supply of deceased-donor organs and the pressures that have led the OPTN to become involved in live-donor policy. Chapter 5 presents the extended controversy over OPTN rules for the allocation of livers. It documents the gradual movement away from local priority in liver allocation in the face of heated and public controversy among OPTN members. More generally, it shows the tensions that can arise in a network between internal and external legitimacy. Chapter 6 explores efforts to address racial disparity in kidney allocation that have resulted in part from the initial adoption of an allocation system placing considerable weight on genetic compatibility between donors and potential recipients. The account reviews a series of incremental changes undertaken over a fifteen-year period to reduce the degree of racial disparity. Chapter 7 considers the capability of the OPTN for making nonincremental change. It looks briefly at one such success, the adoption of a new lung allocation system, and then considers the development of a proposal for a major redesign of the kidney allocation system. In this and the other cases involving changes in allocation policy, the processes of decision making, particularly the uses of information, are set out in some detail to provide an understanding of how this form of governance actually operates. In a nutshell, as summarized in chapter 8, it facilitates evidence-based decision making to an extent that is probably unmatched in any other area of medical policy.

Chapter 9 considers features of the OPTN that appear to contribute to its effectiveness. Specifically, it discusses eight features: professional engagement, continuity, meaningful stakes, decision making by voting, specialization with consultation, transparency, data for creating evidence, and strategic oversight. Stepping beyond the usual bounds of social science, this final chapter also sketches incremental and more radical applications of OPTN-style governance. It proposes marginal changes that would transform the advisory body being created to promote interoperable electronic medical records into a private rulemaker. It then turns to the creation of a private rulemaker to introduce incentives for the implementation of evidence-based assessment of surgical procedures as a mechanism for promoting effective practice and controlling the rate of increase in Medicare expenditures for physician services.

2

Balancing Values, Expertise, and Interests

The governance of the U.S. health care system is exceptionally complex and incorporates a great variety of institutional arrangements. Many of these regulate and subsidize market activity. Others seek to provide bureaus with the information and expertise they require to carry out their tasks but cannot easily collect or maintain in isolation from stakeholders. One goal of this chapter is to provide an overview of the ways these arrangements mediate values, interests, and expertise in medical governance. Another is to introduce and place in context the particular form of medical governance—private rulemaking—that is the empirical focus of this book.

To be sure, the debate over universal health insurance in the United States often rhetorically poses a stark choice between only two forms of governance: market allocation, in which consumers make decisions about health care, versus government allocation, in which bureaucrats make them. Each caricatures governance, claiming extreme forms that would be untenable. Relatively few medical decisions actually follow the ideal model of consumer choice—health insurers, both private and public, generally serve as intermediaries between health care providers and less than perfectly informed consumers. Although the federal government plays major roles in funding and regulating health care, bureaus generally do not make decisions in isolation from medical professionals and other stakeholders. Unregulated market allocation proves undesirable because of fundamental market failures that plague medical care as well as the unacceptable distributional outcomes it would produce. Bureaucratic governance suffers from generic government failures heightened by rapid changes in medical knowledge and technology. Nonetheless, briefly considering these unviable extremes is a useful thought experiment for setting the stage for considering practical options for medical governance.

Governance by Unregulated Market

Imagine a world in which the government played no role in medical care. Doctors or others claiming medical expertise would likely sell services for a fee. Based on the prices of offered services, patients would purchase those services they perceived as offering them benefit in excess of price. Competition among medical care suppliers would drive prices to the minimum levels necessary to compensate them for their time and other costs. With consumers purchasing only services that offer benefits in excess of price, society would realize the largest possible gain. Or would it?

Welfare economists have long recognized a number of ways that market allocation fails to maximize social benefits (for an overview, see Weimer and Vining 2005). That is, some alternative allocation to the one prevailing in the market equilibrium would provide even larger social benefits. Four market failures, three of which are related to uncertainty, are particularly relevant to this stylized market: information asymmetry between providers and patients, incomplete insurance as a relevant missing market, and the public good nature of information about medical procedures and those who provide them.

Information asymmetry occurs when one party has information that, if fully revealed, would change the other party's participation in a transaction. In a seminal article on medical economics, Kenneth Arrow (1963) recognizes the important role of uncertainty, including information asymmetry, in the market for medical care. The providers of medical care enjoy an informational advantage about the potential benefits and risks of the services they offer relative to most of their patients, many of whom will be facing the illness for the first time and will therefore be unable to draw on personal experience. The informational advantage involves both the generic service being provided and the skill of the provider. Further, medical providers may have a financial incentive to encourage patients to purchase services that offer less benefit than their price.

In the welfare economics framework, efficient market allocation requires that all relevant goods be traded in markets. Arrow (1963) identifies the market for insurance as fundamentally relevant to medical care. People generally do not know whether they will become ill at any given time or the expenses they might incur should they become so. Although there is a market for health insurance, it is incomplete for a number of reasons. (A more appropriate term would be medical insurance, but in common usage this term refers to insurance for the services physicians deliver rather than to the more comprehensive coverage that includes hospital services.) Most important, moral hazard and adverse selection make it impossible for insurers to offer full coverage to all people at even approximately actuarially fair prices. Moral hazard occurs when people change their risk-related behavior on the basis of their insurance coverage. For example, one might floss less often when one's dental expenses are covered by insurance. Adverse selection, information asymmetry favoring the buyers of insurance, makes it difficult for insurers to develop homogeneous risk pools. Insurers typically set premiums much lower for coverage sold to groups organized for employment or some other reason largely unrelated to the health of the members than for coverage sold directly to individuals. These problems either result in the absence of coverage for some people, such as those with existing adverse health conditions, or the availability of coverage with large deductibles and copayments that force policy holders to continue to bear substantial risk.

The third important market failure, which health economists generally give less attention, is the public goods nature of information about the efficacy and risk of various kinds of medical care. Nonrivalry (consumption by one does not preclude consumption by others) and nonexclusion (access cannot be economically denied to potential users even if they do not contribute to supply) characterize pure public goods. Information of all sorts fits this definition. For example, all those with a particular disease can benefit from information about the effectiveness of a treatment for it. Once that information is produced, it is usually not practical for those who produce it to keep it confidential; consequently, they cannot capture the full benefit of the efforts they make to provide it. Few private actors are therefore willing to bear the costs of collecting the systematic data on treatments and outcomes necessary to implement socially desirable levels of evidence-based medicine.

The fourth market failure arises because market supply may also involve various sorts of externalities, or situations in which people do not bear the full costs or benefits of their actions. For example, those who pay to be vaccinated against a communicable disease confer a benefit on those who are not vaccinated. It is thus possible that vaccination would not be a desirable choice from an individual's perspective but would be from society's. Behaviors related to health also often impose costs on others. For instance, those who abuse alcohol may place the health of others at risk when they drive under the influence, those with mental illnesses may impose costs on others when they fail to medicate, those who engage in risky sexual behavior may spread sexually transmitted diseases, and those who smoke cigarettes may threaten the health of those around them with secondhand smoke.

In addition to these market failures, which bring into question the efficiency of unregulated market supply, most observers would also be concerned about distributional consequences. Market allocation would price some people, who were unlucky enough to suffer serious illnesses, out of medical care necessary for recovery or even survival. Families unable to afford health insurance would be particularly vulnerable to such catastrophic events. One need not embrace egalitarian values to be concerned about such losses. Belief in the intrinsic value of human life might lead one to consider denying basic medical care socially undesirable.

Of course, it would be a mistake to think that there would be no nongovernmental responses to the shortcomings of unregulated market allocation. Secondary markets for information about medical care would likely arise to mitigate to some extent the information asymmetry problems (Vining and Weimer 1988). Professional societies, such as the American Medical Association, would form to set minimum standards for medical providers and certify those who met the standards. However, once established, these societies would have an economic incentive to limit membership and to attempt to block practice by competing types of medical care providers. Insurers would seek to eliminate services that were not cost-effective and providers who were not competent. Hospitals would create formularies and professional societies would create drug compendia, as they did in the United States before federal pharmaceutical regulation, to weed out some of the least effective and most dangerous drugs. Various organizations would provide medical services to their members, as did fraternal organizations in the United States during the first half of the twentieth century (Beito 2000). Religious and other organizations would create not-for-profit hospitals to provide considerable charitable care. Many people would voluntarily contribute to these efforts, as well as to research sponsored by organizations created to fight particular diseases.

What would medical care look like today had we preserved an unregulated market system by not subsidizing employment-based health insurance through the tax code, by not creating Medicare and Medicaid, by not regulating pharmaceuticals and medical devices, and by not investing huge sums of federal money in medical research? One can speculate that prices would be lower, but largely because fewer people would have health insurance that enabled them to afford extensive medical care. The absence of federal support for research would have resulted in slower advances in medical knowledge and technology and therefore fewer treatment options. Almost certainly, the medical care industry would be a smaller fraction of the economy than it is today.

Even if one views this counterfactual as preferable to the current system of medical governance, the great variety of existing public interventions in medical care initiated in the latter half of the twentieth century prevent a return to an unregulated market. To what extent do consumers make market choices in our current system of medical care? The very wealthy or those with traditional indemnity health insurance plans who live in urban areas with numerous providers have many choices. However, it may be difficult for them to compare prices and quality across the readily available choices. The increasingly common managed care health plans typically restrict choice to a predetermined set of medical care providers. Those of moderate or low income who do not have health insurance have severely restricted choice, primarily limited to acute care available through emergency rooms. In this environment, much of the competition in the medical care market is among health insurance providers for desirable enrollees, or more typically group accounts, rather than among medical care providers attempting to lure patients with attractive combinations of price and quality. A number of observers, most prominently Michael Porter and Elizabeth Olmsted Teisberg, question the value of the former sort of competition and argue for the desirability of having more of the latter (2006).

Governance through Bureaucratic Supply

The canonical bureau consists of government-paid employees organized in a hierarchy to apply expertise in the exercise of authority over some domain of activity—in other words, Max Weber's legal-rational bureaucracy (1947), or at least that bureaucracy as a way to achieve social ends as determined within a pluralistic polity (Constas 1958). In theory, bureaus can recruit appropriately skilled personnel to produce or oversee provision of socially desired goods, such as medical care itself or information about the efficacy of alternative types of medical care, that might not be provided by an unregulated or unsubsidized market. They usually offer these goods at zero, or some administered, price to the general public or more targeted groups. For example, public schools provide free primary and elementary schooling to the children of parents living in their districts, and the Department of Veterans Affairs operates hospitals and its personnel provide medical services, often at zero price, to those discharged from active military duty. Thus, when the market fails to supply reliably an efficient quantity, desirable quality, or acceptable distribution of some good, one public policy alternative is either production or purchase of the good by a bureau funded from tax revenue. The bureau could produce medical care through the physicians it employs; it could also purchase care from private providers, either for specific populations as with Medicaid and Medicare or for the general population through a single-payer system as in the Canadian provinces. In either case, the bureau would have to decide what is to be supplied and at what price and to whom.

Just as unregulated markets can fail in generic ways, so too can bureaus. Unlike firms selling in competitive markets, bureaus with monopolies not only restrict their clients' choices but also cannot rely on prices to signal the value consumers place on various goods. Instead, they must rely on queuing or complaints to learn about consumer satisfaction and must resort to surveys or indirect analysis to assess consumer value. The absence of competition denies the bureau a direct benchmark, its profitability and that of its competitors, for judging its performance. The absence of competitive pressures blunts incentives for improving technology and the bureaus are thus unlikely to be dynamically efficient. The design of bureaus to ensure accountability to the public further hinders their efficiency through restrictions on the discretion of bureau managers in terms of hiring and motivating employees, using financial and other resources, and accessing capital markets. Further, the incentives for efficiency-enhancing oversight by multiple political overseers are generally weaker than for those who can gain profit from contesting the ownership of for-profit organizations (Vining and Weimer 1990).

Just as an unregulated market for medical care is an unpalatable and unrealistic alternative, so too is the direct production of medical care for the general population by a bureaucracy. Perhaps a bureau as a single payer to private medical care providers is a more realistic alternative. In this role, and less extreme ones, the bureau would primarily be concerned with the production of rules to govern the availability and quality of care. Consequently, an assessment of rulemaking by public agencies is a natural starting point for surveying medical governance arrangements.

Public Rulemaking

In the United States, executive agencies issue rules relevant to health, safety, environmental quality, and other policy areas under authorities delegated by Congress through various statutes. Federal agencies exercise these quasi-legislative authorities under general guidelines established by the Administrative Procedure Act of 1946 (Public Law 79-404), which was intended to ensure procedural fairness in the regulatory process, as well as under the specific provisions of their enabling statutes. With only a few exceptions, the act requires agencies to publish proposed rules and accept comments from the public for a period of no fewer than thirty days before publishing final rules in the *Federal Register* to be incorporated into the *Code of Federal Regulations*. Rules may be challenged in federal courts if they violate procedural due process or are not supported by substantial evidence. Because of these requirements and the opportunity for disgruntled parties to seek judicial review, the regulatory process often moves slowly.

Federal regulatory agencies, whether embedded within the hierarchies of executive departments, such as the regulatory offices of the U.S. Environmental Protection Agency (EPA) or the U.S. Food and Drug Administration (FDA), or established as independent commissions with majority rule voting by appointed boards of directors, such as the Federal Communications Commission and the Federal Trade Commission, hire and fire according to civil service rules administered by the Office of Personnel Management. These rules slow the hiring process, sometimes discouraging qualified people from pursuing federal careers. Efforts to create fair salary structures across all federal executive agencies make it difficult for agencies to compete with the private sector for employees with particularly rare skills that have not been recognized in established job classifications. These factors make it particularly difficult for agencies to convince active researchers to trade laboratory for regulatory work.

Even when effective leadership and favorable organizational cultures enable agencies to develop substantial in-house expertise relevant to their general regulatory missions, the serendipity of scientific research and technological development may thrust new issues, demanding very specialized expertise, onto the regulatory agenda. By their very nature, new scientific and technological claims tend to be controversial, denying agencies the luxury of simply observing a consensus among relevant experts. When scientific findings and new technologies raise health and safety concerns, it may not be politically possible or socially desirable for the agency to wait for a consensus to develop. It is not surprising, then, that agencies seek out ways to obtain the advice of those with the specialized knowledge needed to supplement general intramural expertise.

Tapping Extramural Expertise: Advisory Panels

The federal government has a long history of using advisory panels. George Washington convened a number of commissions, including the Whiskey Rebellion Commission (B. Smith 1992, 14), and as early as 1842 Congress sought to control executive branch expenditures on advisory commissions (Croley and Funk 1997, 453). As science and industry became more entangled with executive agencies during World War II and the Cold War that followed, the number of advisory committees grew substantially. Research sponsors, facing the problem of having less information about the integrity and productivity of researchers than the research community, came to rely heavily on advisory and peer-review panels in their evaluation of research proposals (Guston 2000). For example, by the mid-1980s, the National Institutes of Health had created sixty-five study sections that met three times a year to review research proposals (Barke 1986, 83). The role of advisory committees in rulemaking increased with the economic interventions of the New Deal. The demands for scientific and technical advice increased further with the expanding scope of federal health and safety regulation beginning in 1962 with the Kefauver-Harris amendments to the Food, Drug, and Cosmetics Act, which required the FDA to assess the efficacy of all drugs approved for marketing between 1938 and 1962 (Friedman 1978, 206). In 1970, a congressional report estimated that approximately three thousand committees of all types were advising the federal government (Croley and Funk 1997, 460).

Congressional concerns about the large number of advisory committees, their expense, inconsistencies in their use, and lack of balance in their memberships, resulted in legislation establishing a new framework in 1972 (B. Smith 1992, 22). The Federal Advisory Committee Act (Public Law 92-463) put in place the current legal framework for the establishment and use of groups assembled to offer advice or recommendations to the federal government. Its provisions fall into three broad areas (Croley and Funk 1997, 461–65).

First, it addresses unnecessary use of advisory committees. Standing committees of Congress are required to review the advisory committees serving the agencies they oversee, and to determine whether the roles of proposed advisory committees could be played by agency personnel or existing committees. To encourage agencies to reassess their needs for existing committees, the act requires that committees be rechartered every two years unless otherwise specified by statute. As a result, the number of committees fell from 1,439 in 1972 to 816 in 1978 (Petracca 1986, 85), but rose gradually to 915 in 2007 (GAO 2008, 1).

Second, the act addresses formation of advisory committees whose members share particular views, such as committees consisting solely of members drawn from an industry. The act requires Congress to seek fair balance in terms of the points of view represented among the members of committees it authorizes, and the act has been interpreted through subsequent regulations to place the same requirement on agencies. These regulations also require agencies to announce their intentions to create advisory committees in the *Federal Register*, to assess potential conflicts of interest, to monitor committees closely by maintaining control over committee agendas and meetings, and to ensure that an appropriate federal employee be present at every committee meeting. Studies of advisory committees both before (Friedman 1978) and after (Petracca 1986) the 1972 act raise concerns about undue industry influence relative to that of consumers. Nonetheless, based on a detailed assessment of the National Drinking Water Advisory Council, Steven Balla and John Wright argue that agencies give weight to interest group endorsements of committee nominees so that the pattern of interest representation on the committee mirrors that in Congress (2001, 811). More generally, interest group endorsements provide clear indications to members of Congress of the policy preferences of appointees, perhaps facilitating fire-alarm oversight (McCubbins and Schwartz 1984).

Third, the act addresses openness. In the spirit of the Freedom of Information Act, which preceded it in 1966 (Public Law 89-487), and the Government in the Sunshine Act, which followed it in 1976 (Public Law 94-409), the Federal Advisory Committee Act requires that advisory committee meetings not only be announced in advance in the *Federal Register* but also, with a few exceptions, be open to the public. Detailed minutes of meetings must be kept and made available to the public for inspection and copying. This transparency contrasts starkly with the largely hidden processes through which proposed rules are developed internally by the sponsoring agencies.

Agencies continue to rely heavily on advisory committees. For example, a 1992 study by an Institute of Medicine (IOM) committee found that the FDA used forty-one standing technical advisory committees that helped with the evaluation of specific drugs, biological products, and medical devices, and, especially with respect to biological products, helped the agency set general guidelines (Rettig, Early, and Merrill 1992). Committees dealing with controversial issues may draw audiences in the hundreds, including representatives of drug sponsors, their competitors, investors, and the media, suggesting that participants view committee recommendations as influential (Rettig, Early, and Merrill 1992, 34).

FDA decisions concerning the marketing of pharmaceuticals have been frequently criticized by the press, scholars, and congressional oversight committees since implementation of the 1962 Kefauver-Harris amendments (Public Law 87-781), which gave the agency responsibility for assessing the efficacy as well as the safety of new drugs. More recently, the criticisms have included charges that the FDA has inappropriately allowed political ideology to enter its decision-making processes (Steinbrook 2004). One prominent case, for example, is the failure of the FDA for an extended period to approve Plan B, a morning-after pill, for over-the-counter sales despite strong advice from advisory committees to do so. It has led to resignations of agency staff and advisory committee members (Davidoff 2006) as well as senators blocking or delaying the confirmation of FDA commissioners. Although science and medicine under the most recent Bush administration seems more politicized than in the past, we should also remember that one of the first executive orders of the Clinton administration instructed the secretary of Health and Human Services to assess initiatives to promote RU 486, a drug combination that induces abortion (Jackman 2002).

Although notorious cases provide warnings about the range of possible outcomes, the handling of mundane cases is at least as important from the perspective of institutional design. Unfortunately, almost no research has focused on relating advisory committee advice to agency decision making across representative sets of cases. One exception is a study of the impact of FDA advisory committees on the approval of new drug applications (Lavertu and Weimer 2008). For 169 committee votes taken from 1997 through 2006, the percentage of committee members voting yes significantly, both substantively and statistically, increased the probability of FDA approval and, for those applications approved, the speed with which they were approved. Looking across all new drug applications, it appeared that referral to committees increased the average approval time overall, but reduced it for the applications involving the highest levels of uncertainty. In terms of the politicization of the FDA, the study found a lower rate of referral to committees during the Bush than the Clinton administration, but no difference in the influence of committee votes on agency actions. The study did not address possible changes in the makeup of the committees, however.

How important are conflicts of interest among committee members? A study of FDA advisory committee meetings between 2001 through 2004 finds that for almost three-quarters of meetings at least one committee member revealed a conflict of interest and recusal by that person was rare (Laurie et al. 2006). The same study found that conflicts appeared to have some influence on votes, but none were pivotal in terms of the majority position—nonetheless, as the percentage voting yes, rather than the presence of a majority, seems to influence FDA decisions (Lavertu and Weimer 2008), the conflict of interest may be relevant even if not pivotal. More generally, a recent IOM study concluded that concerns about the independence of committee members had cast a "shadow on the trustworthiness" of the scientific advice received by the agency, and recommended that the "FDA establish a requirement that a substantial majority of the members of each advisory committee be free from significant financial involvement with companies whose interests may be affected by the committee's deliberations" (Baciu, Stratton, and Burke 2007, 10).

The FDA committees support the agency's basic tasks of reviewing new drug and device applications within the existing policy framework. In many circumstances, agencies, or sometimes Congress, turn to ad hoc committees of experts to advise on larger policy issues. The committees can be organized by either the relevant agency or, when the independence of the committee is a concern, an external body.

The most well-developed example of the agency use of ad hoc committees in medical governance is the Consensus Development Program of National Institutes of Health, which was begun in 1977. Panels of experts are convened for a conference of two or three days to assess the evidence relevant to medical controversies and communicate the findings to medical practitioners and other interested parties. During the conference, the panelists function much like a jury, hearing evidence presented by speakers and discussants. In the first thirty years of the program, more than 140 consensus development conferences were held, on topics ranging from breast cancer screening to the health benefits of pets. Assessments of the early operation of the panels raised concern about bias in the selection of questions to be addressed and of panelists (Wortman, Vinokur, and Sechrest 1988), behind-the-scenes political influence on the choice of questions (Markle and Chubin 1987), the lack of impact of panel findings on medical practice (Lomas 1991), and the perceptions of participants (Ferguson and Sherman 2001). Dissemination efforts have increased in recent years and findings are routinely published in major medical journals. Evidence also indicates that the findings have influenced research funding (Portnoy et al. 2007).

The findings of the panels have not always been without controversy. A particularly heated dispute surrounded the 1997 panel on the question of whether women age forty to forty-nine should receive regular mammography screening (National Institute of Medicine 1997). The panel failed to reach consensus. Its interpretation of evidence was severely criticized (Kopans 1999) and its finding against screening women in their forties was rejected by the American Cancer Society. The barriers to consensus seem to have been related to the difficulties of interpreting and conveying risks and disagreement about how to take account of costs (Ransohoff and Harris 1997), considerations routinely encountered in developing and assessing policy.

Some scholars have questioned the wisdom of creating expectations of consensus for advisory groups. Although consensus is often strategically valuable in allowing policy makers to take findings as established, theoretical work applying the Condorcet jury theorem suggests that decisions based on super majorities better aggregate the information held by individual committee members than a requirement for consensus does (Gabel and Shipan 2004; for a general survey of the game theoretic literature on committees, see also Gerling et al. 2005). Further, structuring processes to reach a consensus may result in over-simplifying complexity and conflict with openness and accountability (Spielman 2003).

The most prominent mechanism at the federal level for Congress or an agency to obtain independent advice is a contract with the National Academy of Sciences calling for it to appoint and manage an ad hoc committee of experts. The primary mission of the National Academy of Sciences, which was chartered by Abraham Lincoln in 1863, is to advise the federal government on matters of science and technology. Its membership and functions expanded substantially during World War I with the creation of the National Research Council and again in 1970 with the creation of the Institute of Medicine and the National Academy of Engineering. These four units are collectively referred to as the National Academies. Most of the funding of these units, which pays for permanent staffs to support committee work, comes through federal contracts for specifically requested studies. Its elected members, which include the most prominent American scientists, engineers, and medical researchers, often serve with other recruited experts as anonymous peer reviewers for committee work. Its prestige allows it to recruit highly qualified experts to do the pro bono committee work and its reports are widely viewed as credible. However, despite the extensive use of volunteer time, producing the reports is costly. Also, because of the careful processes in assembling committees, seeking consensus, and reviewing findings, as well as delays introduced by agency funding processes, producing reports within short time frames is usually not feasible (Ahearne and Blair 2003).

Congressional requirements for studies of controversial issues by the National Academies written into agency appropriations is one indication of their credibility. For example, as discussed in chapter 5, major controversy between the Department of Health and Human Services (HHS) and the United Network for Organ Sharing (UNOS) over the geographic basis of organ allocation prompted Congress to mandate that HHS fund, before they were finalized, a study of the regulations by the IOM. Between 1991 and 2001, Congress mandated 191 studies by the Academies (Morgan and Peha 2003, appendix 2). Agencies also request National Academy studies without being directed to do so by Congress.

State legislatures are generally less able to draw on independently sponsored advisory committees. One notable exception is the California Health Benefits Review Program (CHBRP), which is administered by the University of California. It was established in 2002 by the California legislature out of concern for the increasing cost of health insurance resulting from coverage mandates. It consists of a small full-time staff, recruitment of faculty to conduct specific analyses, and a national advisory board of experts and stakeholders not directly affected by the proposed mandates. An assessment of the CHBRP by Thomas Oliver and Rachel Friedman Singer (2006) finds that its reports guided policy design but also provided political ammunition. Oliver and Singer also find that, though the review process appeared to reduce the number of new mandates, it was generally supported by both proponents and opponents of mandates.

How well do committees advising regulatory agencies on larger policy issues perform? Sheila Jasanoff sought to answer this question through case studies of a number of advisory committees used by the EPA and the FDA (1990, 230–36). She concludes that a strict separation of science from politics is generally impractical. Further, attempts to maintain a strict separation often produce more conflict than explicit integration of science into policymaking. Advisory committees seem to be most effective when they facilitate negotiation among those with divergent views, both scientific and nonscientific, and when they are successful in defining sharp boundaries around what can be considered as scientific issues and, therefore, are not subject to challenge by nonscientists. Jasanoff sees the primary problem in the effective use of advisory committees as not so much guarding against the danger that a narrow scientific view will dominate the regulatory process, but rather as finding better ways for the agencies to "harness the collective expertise of scientific community so as to advance the public interest" (1990, 250).

Bruce L. R. Smith reaches similar conclusions based on his study of science advising at the Department of Defense, the EPA, the Department of Energy, the National Aeronautics and Space Administration, and the Department of State (1992). He notes a paradox facing the advisor: "He or she must become a true insider to accomplish anything; but in doing so the adviser may lose the fresh view, detachment, and outsider qualities that are urgently required" (193).

Overall, these accounts suggest that advisory committees play an important, if imperfect, role in supplementing agency expertise. The most effective committees appear to be those that can reach at least a near consensus on answers to clearly delineated scientific or technical questions and relate these answers to the immediate policy issues facing agencies. Yet integrating expertise into policy requires an understanding of the various value trade-offs confronting policymakers. Can committees drawn solely on the basis of their scientific and technical expertise have enough understanding of these trade-offs to shape effective advice? Can committees drawn to include divergent points of view to facilitate a sophisticated understanding of value trade-offs (say, through the inclusion of stakeholder interests) enjoy enough credibility and the possibility of achieving near consensus to have an independent effect on the policy process? If a committee included both credible scientific and technical expertise and representation of all stakeholders, would it be a desirable forum for decision making? The first two questions make clear the tension in the use of expert committees in public rulemaking; an affirmative answer to the third question suggests a more radical alternative, private rulemaking, in which the stakeholders actually determine the content of rules.

Increasing Rapidity? Co-opting Stakeholders through Negotiated Rulemaking

The increased involvement of the federal government in the economy that began in the New Deal and extended in scope with the creation of new regulatory agencies in the early 1970s, such as the Occupational Safety and Health Administration and the EPA in 1970, and the Consumer Products Safety Commission in 1972, has been accompanied by an expansion of procedural protections within administrative law for those affected by agency actions.

Specifically, Richard Stewart notes four major doctrinal developments in administrative law by the mid-1970s (1975, 1716). First, the courts adopted an increasingly strong presumption that agency actions were subject to judicial review. Second, the courts recognized a wider range of interests as being entitled to administrative hearings under the due process clause of the constitution. Third, statutes enlarged the classes of interest with legal standing in formal agency processes. Fourth, the courts enlarged the classes of interest with standing to obtain judicial review of agency decisions. In addition to these extensions of recognized interests, the courts gradually abandoned the rational basis test, which gave a presumption to sustaining agency action as long as it had a rational basis, in favor of the hard look standard of review, which requires agencies to consider closely all the relevant issues involved in the action (Harter 1982, 11). More recently, Supreme Court decisions have signaled somewhat more deference to agency discretion, especially with respect to their interpretation of scientific evidence in risk assessment (Jasanoff 1995, 84–86). Overall, these doctrinal changes reflect the emergence of a highly adversarial regulatory process over the last forty years.

Beginning in the mid-1970s, various observers of the regulatory process expressed concerns about the disadvantages of adversarial rulemaking. Critics readily acknowledged that an adversarial process could be effective in mobilizing interested parties to gather and present information as well as to detect errors in the information provided by others. At the same time, however, the critics raised concerns about the incentives an adversarial process gives participants to take extreme positions, to conceal information that does not support their positions, to make defensive expenditures on gathering factual information of only marginal value to informing the decision, and to rely too heavily on specialists (lawyers) in the regulatory process (Harter 1982, 19–22). Further, adversarial processes are best for resolving disputes between pairs of parties and are less suitable "for resolving polycentric disputes involving many parties and many possible outcomes... (and) require delicate tradeoffs among competing interests," circumstances that characterize much rule-making (Harter 1982, 20). Adversarial rulemaking was widely perceived as producing poor rules, costing too much, taking too long, and generating too much litigation. Indeed, Cary Coglianese documents how for twenty years prominent practitioners and academics readily accepted and repeated the apocryphal claim that 80 percent of rules produced by the EPA resulted in litigation—there is no empirical basis for the 80 percent figure (1997, appendix D)—and estimates the actual rate to be between 19 and 35 percent, depending on whether the base is all rules or only significant rules under two important statutes (1296–301). Nonetheless, the wide acceptance of the claim suggests that it fit well with observers' perceptions of the highly adversarial nature of the regulatory process.

Concerns about adversarial rulemaking led a number of critics, such as John Dunlop (1976), Peter Shuck (1979), and Philip Harter (1982), to offer negotiated rulemaking as a supplement to the Administrative Procedure Act. Under negotiated rulemaking, the regulatory agency convenes a committee consisting of stakeholders, citizens, and agency staff to draft a proposed rule. The members negotiate among themselves in meetings open to the public. If the members reach a consensus on a rule, then the agency publishes it in appropriate form as a proposed rule in the *Federal Register* for comments as specified in the Administrative Procedure Act. The Negotiated Rulemaking Act of 1990 (Public Law 101-648) and subsequent presidential executive orders have encouraged agencies to make greater use of negotiated rulemaking. Proponents argued that, by involving stakeholders in the drafting process, negotiated rulemaking would produce rules more quickly, with greater legitimacy, and with less likelihood of judicial challenge. How has negotiated rulemaking worked in practice?

In a study of its use by the EPA, Coglianese found little difference between conventional and negotiated rulemaking in terms of calendar time for completing rulemakings or rates of judicial challenge (1997). It appears that the fragility of consensus, especially in the face of subsequent revisions of the rule in formal drafting and as a result of public comments and Office of Management and Budget review, is one source of litigation—even small changes during formalization can unravel the consensus. Another source is organizations excluded from formal participation, either because they were not selected to participate or because they became interested only as the negotiations proceeded.

Laura Langbein and Cornelius Kerwin conducted extensive surveys of participants in eight negotiated and six conventional EPA rulemakings (2000). Like Coglianese, they discovered little difference in terms of the rates of judicial challenge between conventional and negotiated rulemaking. They did find differences between the types of rulemaking in terms of the perceptions of participants, however. In particular, those participating in negotiated rulemaking showed greater satisfaction with the content of the final rule and the process by which it was produced than those participating in conventional rulemaking. Participants in negotiated rulemaking also reported learning more about the issues involved, but at higher costs to themselves—overall costs of negotiated and conventional rulemaking appear comparable if the time costs of EPA staff are also taken into account (Freeman and Langbein 2000).

A broader study suggests that, other things equal, consensual rulemaking (either negotiated rulemaking or the use of advisory committees) slows down rulemaking. Steven

Balla and John Wright analyzed 170 major rulemakings completed between March 1996 and June 1999 (2003). They found that, taking into account the tendency of agencies to select rulemakings of shorter duration (selection bias) for handling through negotiation, negotiated rulemaking appeared to increase the time from proposed to final rules. Further, they found that the use of advisory committees also slowed down rulemaking.

Although negotiated rulemaking produces rules neither more quickly nor with less likelihood of being challenged than those produced through conventional rulemaking, it does appear to offer some benefits in terms of participants' more favorable perception of the regulatory process and their learning about the issue at hand and those related to it. Like negotiated rulemaking, private rulemaking involves participation by stakeholders. Unlike it, private rulemaking involves ongoing interactions among stakeholders and produces de facto final rules through voting rather than proposed rules by consensus.

Private Rulemaking

Although private rulemaking is a rather rare alternative to its public counterpart, private standard-setting is a common supplement for, or complement to, public standard-setting. Many private organizations in the United States, including Underwriters Laboratories, the American Society for Testing and Materials, and the American National Standards Institute, maintain many thousands of standards. To assess the relative effectiveness of private and public standard-setting, Ross Cheit conducted case studies in four substantive areas in which plausible comparisons could be made (1990). Although public standard-setting appeared to enjoy some advantages, such as greater capacity for collecting information about risks from the actual use of products, private standard-setting appeared to offer a more flexible and adaptive process:

> The case studies suggest that there are significant evolutionary differences between public and private standard-setters, differences that indicate several previously unrecognized advantages of the private sector. In short, private standards-setting is prospective and ongoing, while public efforts are usually corrective and singular. Private standards-setters tend to intervene relatively early in the life cycle of an issue, adjusting the standard subsequently over time. Public standards-setters, by contrast, are likely to get involved later, often after a major disaster, adopting a "one-shot" standard without the benefit of subsequent adjustments. (Cheit 1990, 202)

Giandomenico Majone sketches a similar comparison of standard setting by the European Commission and private or semi-private standardization bodies in Europe (1996, 23–26).

Private standard-setting has been common in medical governance. For example, many professional associations set standards for certification of medical specialties. They can also have broader impact. For instance, consider managed care. Since 1991 the nonprofit National Committee on Quality Assurance, with encouragement and support from corporate purchasers of employee health plans, has been developing the Health Plan and

Employers Data Information Set (HEDIS) as a way to assess the quality of care health maintenance and other managed care organizations provide. By 1994, three-quarters of managed care organizations used at least some HEDIS measures (Physician Payment Review Commission 1997, 150–51; Gormley and Weimer 1999, 180–81). The adoption of HEDIS continues to expand as states increasingly require private accreditation under their contracts with managed care organizations for the provision of services to Medicaid participants.

On the surface, this comparison of public and private standard-setting may not seem relevant to the comparison of private and public rulemaking, because the private standards by themselves do not directly constrain behavior. Private standards gain force, however, in a number of ways. First, they may become legally binding by being adopted by regulatory agencies. An extreme example is the wholesale adoption of private standards by the Occupational Safety and Health Administration at its inception (Mendeloff 1979). Second, they may gain commercial force by becoming common requirements in private contractual relations. For example, construction contracts often require that the materials used meet standards set by Underwriters Laboratories or other private standard-setters. Third, they may gain force under civil law by reducing vulnerability to tort for those who adhere to them. Fourth, private standards applied to organizations through accreditation processes may gain force when accreditation becomes a requirement for participation in government programs (Havighurst 1994). Finally, governments and other third-party payers may reimburse accredited service providers at higher rates. For example, a number of states reimburse day care centers certified by the National Association for the Education of Children at higher rates to reward the higher quality thought to be associated with accreditation (William T. Gormley Jr., personal communication to the author, August 1, 2008).

Private standard-setting uses stakeholder expertise directly in an ongoing process of drafting and revising the substantive content of standards that influence behavior and sometimes effectively constrain it. Private rulemaking also directly uses stakeholder expertise in an ongoing process of drafting and revising the substantive content of rules that are de facto binding.

Private regulation in various forms has always had a significant role in U.S. political economy. Many states rely heavily on private organizations in setting the conditions for the certification and licensing of those who wish to practice professions such as law and medicine (Hollings and Pike-Nase 1997). Industries often form organizations to engage in self-regulation to weed out firms that attempt to gain market share with low-cost but low-quality products, to head off threats of public regulation, or to establish defenses against legal negligence. Professionals, such as industrial hygienists and accountants, who work within firms, often bring norms of practice that constrain managerial discretion to achieve goals that might otherwise be addressed through public regulation. Professions may also take the initiative to regularize their environments in ways that facilitate good practice. For example, the American College of Surgeons began the hospital standardization program in 1919, shifting the emphasis in hospital management from hotel services to patient care based on their tacit knowledge, or what has been called the orderly use of experience (Rees 2008, 2). Philosophers Harry Collins and Robert Evans liken the acquisition of tacit knowledge to "learning natural language—something attained by interactive immersion in the way of life of the culture rather than by extended study of dictionaries and grammars or their equivalents" (2007, 23). For example, not only do surgeons learn their craft through practice and participation in surgical teams (who would want to go under the knife of someone who had only read about doing surgery?), they are also immersed in interactions with patients, other surgeons and medical professionals, professional societies, and administrators. It is through these contexts that they develop relevant knowledge about good surgery that could not be distilled in a functional set of formal rules. Much of their expertise is thus tacit.

Concern about the undesirable consequences of the adversarial nature of agency rulemaking, which led to calls for negotiated rulemaking, has been matched by concern about the consequences of the adversarial nature of the relationship between the inspectorate that implements regulations and those being regulated. Eugene Bardach and Robert Kagan analyzed the problems that arise from the standardization required if public regulation is to satisfy requirements of due process and equal treatment before the law in the face of the "diversity, complexity, and fluidity of the real world" (1982, 92). Standardization inevitably creates enforcement that appears unreasonable. Reactions to the unreasonableness create a vicious circle: "When regulatory systems seem to act unreasonably, businessmen react defensively. Enforcement officials, when challenged, respond with enhanced mistrust and legalism. Businessmen become still more resentful and retaliate with various forms of noncooperation and resistance" (107). Bardach and Kagan see private regulation as avoiding this vicious circle and therefore deserving of greater consideration in the choice of policy instruments for achieving regulatory goals (1982).

A particular form of private regulation, private rulemaking, is the empirical focus of this volume. It has three essential elements. First, it is carried out by a nongovernmental organization that includes representation of the major stakeholders. Second, the organization has a charter, under either statute or administrative delegation, to formulate the substantive content of rules under a specified voting procedure. Third, either the rules have immediate effect by virtue of the membership within the organization of those whose actions are necessary to implement them, or, if the organization is accountable to a regulatory agency, the agency generally accepts the substance of the rules through either passive acquiescence or routine approval

Table 2–1 emphasizes the differences between conventional public rulemaking and private rulemaking in terms of the use of expertise and stakeholder involvement in designing rules. The extreme upper left cell describes conventional rulemaking, in which the agency provides the necessary expertise for developing the rule in-house and involves stakeholders either informally or through a notice and comment process. The extreme lower right cell describes private rulemaking, in which there is a full delegation over substantive content to a body of self-governing stakeholders. Negotiated rulemaking involves stakeholders directly in developing rules, though the agency has responsibility for drafting them. If the agency chooses to turn to an external body, such as the National Academies, or is forced to do so by Congress, the cells show the addition to the regulatory process of the input from commissioned panels. Finally, as illustrated later in governance arrangements like the Advisory Committee on Immunization Practices, a panel chartered by the agency or Congress may be supervised by the agency under the Advisory Committee Act but have de facto, or even de jure, authority to make rules in some specified circumstances.

Table 2–1   **Regulatory Forms**

		Stakeholder involvement in rule development		
		Comments on proposed rule	**Direct involvement**	**Full substantive delegation**
Incorporation of external expertise in rule development	Volunteered comments to regulatory docket	Conventional public rulemaking		
	Direct supervision by agency	Conventional rulemaking with advisory panels	Negotiated rulemaking	Chartered panel with authority or hybrid form
	External supervision			Private rulemaking

Source: Author.

In applications of private rulemaking where rules govern the allocation of things of value—such as agricultural quotas (Cave and Salant 1995; Shepard 1986), airport landing slots (Riker and Sened 1991), Internet domain names (Froomkin 2000), and transplant organs—the administrative organization effectively functions as a legalized cartel. When the interests of the dominant stakeholders in the cartel do not well represent the full range of social values, private rulemaking may simply offer a technically efficient way to achieve a socially undesirable allocation. When either all relevant stakeholders are at the table, or many at the table bring professional norms aligned with broader social values to temper private interests, the potential for technical efficiency contributing to social value is much greater. A review of a number of cases of private rulemaking suggests the technical, political, and practical factors relevant to the choice of private rulemaking as an alternative to public rulemaking (Weimer 2006).

Technical Efficiency

One potential reason for the choice of private over public rulemaking is that the former, in some circumstances, offers greater technical efficiency. This is not a claim about the desirability of the selected goals. For example, the higher consumer prices that result from agricultural marketing boards that allocate production quotas are probably not socially desirable. Yet, conditional on the decision to establish production quotas, marketing boards almost certainly offer greater technical efficiency than public rulemaking. Indeed, public rulemaking probably would not be a feasible alternative with plausibly available resources because of the need for current information on local market circumstances.

Private rulemaking is likely to be technically efficient when three conditions hold. First, the major stakeholders participating in the administrative organization have the expertise needed for informed decision making. One rationale for delegating to either agencies or private rulemaking organizations is the need for expertise. In the case of public rulemaking, in-house expertise is supplemented by advisory panels. In the case of private rulemaking, expertise adheres within the organization itself. If rules are to be made by the participating stakeholders, then it is important that those stakeholders collectively have enough expertise to produce technically well-informed rules. Turning things around, when the stakeholders do have the needed expertise, private rulemaking offers the potential advantage of providing a closer connection between experts and decision makers than is typically possible in public rulemaking.

Second, the policy area in which rulemaking takes place involves changing circumstances that demand frequent adjustment of the rules. Paraphrasing Cheit's comparative assessment of standard-setting: "Private rulemaking is prospective and ongoing, [whereas] public rulemaking is usually corrective and singular" (1990, 202). Private rulemaking, because it involves the prominent stakeholders and directly taps their expertise, can move more quickly than its public counterpart. Especially under majority rule voting, decisions, perhaps reflecting compromise to obtain majorities, can be made fairly quickly. The decisions are likely to be incremental changes that can be reversed with additional information. The possibility for providing rapid and flexible responses to new information is the primary source of the technical efficiency of private over public rulemaking.

Third, the tacit knowledge of stakeholders is required to make effective rules. Stakeholders directly involved in the processes being regulated often have firsthand knowledge of conditions on the ground relevant to predicting the consequences of alternative rules. They may know the actual quality of essential data and how that data could be manipulated to game rules. By viewing proposed rules from their own perspective, they may also be able to predict behavioral responses that otherwise would manifest themselves as unintended consequences. Evidence-based expertise may not adequately substitute for this sort of tacit knowledge. Public rulemaking may try to elicit tacit knowledge by including practitioners as well as researchers on its advisory panels during the development of proposed rules and by making special efforts to solicit public comment on them, but these efforts may fail because those with relevant tacit knowledge are not engaged. Private rulemaking provides an opportunity to tap the tacit knowledge of stakeholders throughout the rulemaking process, but especially in developing the rules.

Blame Avoidance

One reason Congress may delegate rulemaking authority is to "to avoid a particularly nettlesome political issue" (Rosenbloom 2000, 135). Private rulemaking offers a potential political advantage over public rulemaking when the choice of rules cannot avoid creating self-identified losers: it removes the content of the rulemaking further from the political agenda. Morris Fiorina notes that shift-the-responsibility models recognize that legislators may wish to move political as well as decision-making costs away from themselves (1982, 46–47). The desire is likely to be strong for issues involving allocation that will unavoidably result in clearly identified losers. Because considerable evidence from cognitive psychology suggests that those who suffer a loss are more likely to perceive it, feel affected by it, and act on that feeling than those who obtain a comparable gain (Kahneman and Tversky 1984), politicians are likely to see the opportunity for claiming credit as more than offset by the risks of accruing blame in situations of zero-sum allocation. In the political calculus of credit claiming and blame avoidance, the latter is likely to dominate (Weaver 1986, 1988). Delegating authority to a regulatory agency tends to shift the focus for debate from the legislative arena to the agency and the courts. In cases involving direct allocation of things of value, however, primary stakeholders who do not receive satisfactory allocations may lobby the legislature or the executive to change the rules, returning the issue to the political agenda. To avoid blame, politicians may seek to insulate themselves from future appeals by delegating rulemaking to nongovernmental organizations with internal procedural rules for resolving, or at least accommodating to some extent, stakeholder conflicts.

The attractiveness of blame avoidance is likely to be particularly large in medical governance, especially when individuals perceive that decisions have direct implications for their own morbidity or mortality. As identifiable victims of proposed rules, those who would be disadvantaged would make dramatic witnesses at congressional hearings and attract human interest media coverage, further raising the prospect that opportunities for politicians to claim credit would be far exceeded by their risks of receiving blame.

Availability

For private rulemaking to be a viable alternative, it must be possible to identify the primary stakeholders and to envision their cooperation within a nongovernmental organization. An existing model of stakeholder cooperation facilitates these tasks. For example, both agricultural marketing boards and the self-regulating organizations in securities regulation, prominent historical examples of private rulemaking, were applications of a general model of delegation to stakeholders used widely during the New Deal era (Jaffe 1937). A well-developed network among stakeholders may provide an adequate model of cooperation, so that the transition to private rulemaking can be accomplished through the creation of a strong network administrative organization.

In addition to the existence of a model of stakeholder cooperation to enable politicians to envision the possibility of private rulemaking, it must actually be possible to enlist all prominent stakeholders. Prominent stakeholders are those with strong enough interests to be potentially willing to invest resources in lobbying and other political activity. They must acquiesce in creating or designating the nongovernmental organization. In doing so, à la McCubbins, Noll, and Weingast (1989), they increase the likelihood that it will produce outcomes acceptable to its political creators. Once the organization is established, its members gain a stake in its preservation because participation in its procedures provides an opportunity to influence, or at least anticipate, policies. Even persistent losers may hesitate to seek a return to public regulation, where there will be greater uncertainty and higher stakes because of the episodic nature of major public rulemakings. An analogy may be drawn with the explanation for the formation and stability of legislative parties John Aldrich advanced (1995): facing unstable, and therefore uncertain, policy outcomes that result from the formation of short-run coalitions around particular issues, legislators may organize parties as long-term coalitions to provide stability in some fundamentally important policy dimension. In the case of private rulemaking organizations, that dimension is collective stakeholder control over the details of the rules.

Stakeholder incentives within private rulemaking organizations differ from those they face in negotiated rulemaking. In negotiated rulemaking, a consensus is sought on the design of a particular rule (a short-run coalition) in the absence of stakeholder concerns about preserving a decision-making body (a long-term coalition). Withholding consensus may stalemate the negotiation; initially given acceptance may be later withdrawn through court challenges. Decision making by majority-rule voting rather than consensus enables private rulemaking organizations to avoid stalemate. The desirability of preserving the organization's authority to make decisions and the desirability of continued participation in the exercise of that authority discourages stakeholders from seeking to overturn specific decisions by moving issues onto the political agenda. Of course, the anticipation of persistent losses on important issues may eventually lead some stakeholders to challenge the long-term coalition.

Private Rulemaking as
Collaborative Governance (on Steroids)

A number of scholars have given attention to various hybrid forms of governance involving direct collaboration among stakeholders and government agencies. These forms have been variously labeled "co-production" (Whitaker 1980), "subcontracting" (Huyse and Parmentier 1990, 259), "mandated full self-regulation" (Gunningham and Rees 1997, 365), or "regulated self-regulation" (Knill and Lehmkuhl 2002, 49–51). The most comprehensive label is collaborative governance.

Chris Ansell and Alison Gash reviewed 137 cases of the use of collaborative governance across a range of policy sectors (2008). Their review leads them to emphasize the importance of there being enough time for a virtuous circle to develop in interaction among participants: face-to-face dialogue and good faith negotiation build trust; trust reinforces commitment to the process, which leads to shared understanding; shared understanding facilitates the achievement of intermediate outcomes, including small wins and joint fact-finding, that in turn encourage further face-to-face dialogue. In terms of institutional design, the possibility for this virtuous circle to take hold requires that the collaboration is the exclusive forum for decision making, participation includes all stakeholders, clear ground rules are established, and processes are transparent.

As an ongoing governance arrangement, private rulemaking provides the continuous interaction needed to develop the virtuous circle. It also can be, and typically is, structured to satisfy the design features Ansell and Gash see as important (2008): an exclusive forum for decision making about the content of some set of rules, broad participation by stakeholders, clearly set-out procedures (including for voting to move rule development

BAKER COLLEGE OF
CLINTON TWP LIBRARY

forward and make decisions in the absence of consensus), and transparency (not just when a rule is proposed but also during its development). It can be thought of as collaborative governance on steroids.

Familiar Medical Governance Arrangements with Attributes of Private Rulemaking

Although private rulemaking as defined here currently is not a common form of medical governance, a number of familiar institutions share some of its attributes. Most important, they influence policy development or implementation with some degree of independence from administrative agencies. That is, they are more than advisory committees to agencies engaged in public rulemaking. A few of these institutions, such as the Oregon Health Services Commission, have received considerable scholarly attention. However, most have not been studied at all from the perspective of governance.

Joint Commission on Accreditation of Healthcare Organizations

Compliance with certain standards as a prerequisite for participation in government programs has been especially important in the health area. In establishing the Medicare program, Congress followed the practice of many insurance companies in allowing participating hospitals to be deemed in compliance with the Medicare conditions of participation if they were accredited by what is now called the Joint Commission on Accreditation of Healthcare Organizations (JCAHO), an organization composed primarily of representatives of associations of health professionals (Jost 1983; Freeman 2000, 610–11). More than 80 percent of hospitals choose to be so deemed for Medicare and Medicaid by JCHAO rather than accredited by the Centers for Medicare and Medicaid Services (GAO 2004, 7). Until 1984 it was a legal requirement rather than an option for psychiatric and tuberculosis hospitals to be accredited by JCAHO (Roberts, Coate, and Redman 1987, 13). Consistent with Cheit's generalization, it appears that JCAHO has continually revised its standards in response to changes in the technology of health care delivery (Jost 1983, 885), the accreditation process is oriented toward helping hospitals comply, and on-site surveys occur every three years; in contrast, the Centers for Medicare and Medicaid Services infrequently revises its standards, seeks to deter noncompliance, and makes site visits much less frequently (Walshe 2003). Nonetheless, there is "little consensus among stakeholders in the JCAHO accreditation process about whether it works or how useful it is, and there is a remarkable absence of empirical evaluation studies that might provide some foundation for a rational debate" (Walshe 2003, 64).

JCAHO has many of the attributes of private rulemaking. Most important, it is a self-governing organization of stakeholders that develops the substantive content of standards. These standards for a time had the force of formal rules for psychiatric and tuberculosis hospitals—JCAHO itself sought to eliminate this regulatory role out of fear that courts would eventually force it to comply with the Administrative Procedures Act and the

Freedom of Information Act (Jost 1983, 888). The standards are currently effectively rules for those hospitals that seek to be deemed accredited by JCAHO rather than by the Centers for Medicare and Medicaid Services.

Oregon Health Services Commission

In 1989 Oregon undertook a multifaceted initiative to reduce the number of its residents who were uninsured. A bold element of the initiative was to confront explicitly the trade-off between the number of people covered by Medicaid and the services covered in the face of a constrained budget. The legislature delegated responsibility to the newly created Health Services Commission to rank diagnostic-treatment pairs in order of priority. A contractor estimated the cost of offering each pair so that the legislature could move down the list with a running tally of how much the accumulated package of services would cost. The legislature imposed on itself a closed rule—to accept or reject the list in its entirety. For example, the 2003 prioritized list had 730 diagnostic-treatment pairs and the legislature funded pairs through 549 initially and then through 546 the following year (Oregon Health Services Commission 2005).

The commission created its first list in 1991, but federal approval through a Medicaid waiver was not granted until 1993 following several revisions to the prioritization methodology. The Oregon Office of Medical Assistance Programs implemented the list in 1994. Since then the list has been revised for each biennial budget.

The Oregon Health Plan, especially the prioritization of services, drew much national attention. One of the objections was that it substituted technocratic expertise for authentic public participation. The process for creating the initial list, however, involved substantial public participation: a telephone survey of residents to provide data for constructing a quality-of-well-being scale specifically for Oregon, forty-seven community meetings, and twelve public hearings (Garland 1992). Since then the commission has continued to consult widely, and, according to one observer, receives good reviews from both producer and consumer groups (Leichter 1999, 151). Tim Tenbensel argues that the commission has been very effective in interpreting and incorporating public values into the prioritization (2002). If we avoid the nirvana fallacy that seems to plague many medical ethicists—comparing public participation in the activities of a real organization, such as the commission, with some ideal of public participation rather than with the sort of participation that would result in decision making by a regulatory agency or legislature—then the commission offers an encouraging view of private rulemaking.

Another line of criticism centered around the initial intention to rank diagnostic-treatment pairs primarily in terms of the quality-of-well-being scale similar to quality-adjusted life-years (La Puma 1992). Because the methodology for applying these scores led to counterintuitive rankings, both because it inappropriately assumed cardinal properties for the scale (Nord 1993) and because of data limitations, the commission adapted its approach to draw on members' expertise to deal with rankings that appeared anomalous (Garland 1992). This prompted some criticism from those who thought that the revised approach reduced the legitimacy of the commission's rankings (Kaplan 1992).

The strongest concerns expressed about the Oregon Health Plan were that it would deny services to the most vulnerable segments of the population. In fact, the cutoffs selected by the legislature appeared primarily to exclude services for which there was little evidence of effectiveness. Further, in implementation, some of these excluded services were actually delivered by the managed care organizations that enrolled the majority of Medicaid participants and others were delivered by physicians as part of the diagnostic process (Bodenheimer 1997; Leichter 1999). As with the concern about methodology, the new criticism became not that the rationing was too strict, but rather that it was not consequential and did not save much money (Oberlander, Marmor, and Jacobs 2001). Nonetheless, the prioritization was a politically important component of the Oregon Health Plan that allowed Oregon to move from an uninsured rate above the national average in 1990 to below the national average today (Leichter 2004). In particular, Lawrence Jacobs, Ted Marmor, and Jonathan Oberlander see the prioritization as having strategic value to reformers by transcending the boundaries among health care actors and providing a forum for continuous negotiation, keeping stakeholders directly engaged for a protracted period (1999, 175). In other words, providing the opportunity for Ansell and Gash's virtuous circle to take hold.

The Health Services Commission is like private rulemaking in that its appointed members make decisions with staff support from a state agency, the Office for Oregon Health Policy and Research, rather than serving as advisors to the agency. These decisions represent a delegation in authority from the legislature to set the agenda for its choice. In other words, the legislature ties its own hands so that it does not have to be involved in making its own comparisons across more than the marginally ranked services—an institutional arrangement conceptually similar to the delegation by Congress of agenda setting authority to the Base Closure and Reallignment Commission beginning in 1990 (Weimer 1992). The members also serve four-year terms, which allows for learning through doing and perhaps contributes to a longer time horizon than if their terms were for only one or two years. Although not appointed by stakeholders, members are broadly representative of the health care sector and consult widely with health care providers. For example, in preparing its Prioritized List of Health Services in the 2003–2005 biennium, the commission thanked six associations for contributing time to its efforts and more than eighty medical practitioners and researchers for reviewing research in their areas of expertise (Oregon Health Services Commission 2005).

Medicare Payment Advisory Commission

Concern about the growing budgetary costs of Medicare Part B, which covers physician services, and the failure of the Reagan administration to answer its requests for reform proposals, led Congress to create the Physician Payment Review Commission in 1985. Its commissioners were appointed by the director of the Office of Technology Assessment in 1986. The commission began issuing reports in 1987 and played a critical role in the adoption of a resource-based physician fee schedule to replace the customary charges system in 1989 (D. Smith 1992).

Thomas Oliver identifies a number of features of the Physician Payment Review Commission that he believes explain its influence (1993). First, its commissioners, appointed on a nonpartisan basis and drawn from medical practice, academia, industry, and relevant organizations, brought high-quality expertise to its tasks, producing information that became generally viewed as independent and evidence-based. Second, it was highly successful in combining analysis with viable proposals for action. Third, by providing sophisticated analysis on a timely basis, it developed close working relationships with both majority and minority staff of the three relevant congressional committees. Fourth, its initial successes resulted in it being progressively assigned more responsibilities so that it effectively became a standing committee with continuing engagement on the collection of related issues. Fifth, it reached out to interest groups, including organizing conferences with stakeholders. Sixth, more so than policy development within regulatory agencies, it operated in the open—deliberations and recommendations were public as were all materials submitted to the commission—creating as sense of accessibility and fairness that further encouraged stakeholder participation.

These factors enabled the commission to remain influential in the ongoing implementation of the resource-based fee schedule. In 1997 Congress created the Medicare Payment Advisory Commission (MedPAC) by merging the Physician Payment Review Commission with the Prospective Payment Assessment Commission, which it had created to advise on the implementation of diagnostic related group payments to hospitals under Medicare Part A. MedPAC, which advises Congress on Medicare issues, has seventeen commissioners appointed for staggered terms by the comptroller general, who heads what is now the Government Accountability Office, on the basis of nominations from stakeholders. The primary formal vehicles for transmitting advice to Congress and the HHS secretary are reports issued in March and June of each year, which include appendices with commissioners' votes on all recommendations. Frequent contacts with congressional staff provide additional avenues for influence. Evidence and analysis support each recommendation. The recommendations themselves are specific. For example, the physician services recommendation in the March 2008 report stated that "Congress should update payments for physician services in 2009 by the projected change in input prices less the Commission's adjustment for productivity growth. The Congress should enact legislation requiring CMS to establish a process for measuring and reporting physician resource use on a confidential basis for a period of two years" (Medicare Payment Advisory Commission 2008, 336).

MedPAC is like a private rulemaker in that it has ongoing involvement in a policy area, makes decisions by voting rather than requiring consensus, and develops the content of proposed rules, although it only makes recommendations that require action by Congress or HHS to take force. Further, it is not self-governing in the sense that the stakeholders nominate, but do not select, commissioners.

Advisory Committee on Immunization Practices

The Advisory Committee on Immunization Practices (ACIP) was established in 1964 to play a traditional advisory role for the HHS and the Centers for Disease Control and

Prevention (CDC) on the best use of vaccines to reduce disease burden. In 1993, however, the Omnibus Budget Reconciliation Act (Public Law 103-66) gave the ACIP rule-making authority with respect to the vaccines, doses, and contraindications provided through the Vaccines for Children Program, an almost $2 billion per year program through which the CDC makes bulk purchases of vaccines for distribution to state and local health agencies.

The ACIP has fifteen voting members who serve four-year terms. The CDC nominates candidate members to provide the committee with relevant expertise and HHS selects members from among those nominated (Pickering 2002). The committee includes ex officio members representing eight federal offices as well as liaison representatives from approximately twenty-five organizations, including professional associations (such as the American Academy of Family Physicians and the American Medical Association), trade associations (such as the Pharmaceutical Research Manufacturers of America and the Biotechnology Industry Organization), and foreign organizations (the Canadian National Advisory Committee on Immunization and the Department of Health of the United Kingdom) (Smith, Snider, and Pickering 2007). Thus the ACIP combines the standard advisory committee structure of appointed voting members and ex officio government members with explicit representation for stakeholder organizations.

The ACIP, which receives staff support from the CDC, meets three times each year to address agenda items solicited from members, liaison representatives, CDC staff, and others. It uses four standing working groups—Adult Immunization Schedule, General Recommendations, Childhood/Adolescent Immunization Schedule, and Influenza Vaccine—as well as approximately ten ad hoc working groups at any time on general topics, such as bioterrorism or vaccination during pregnancy, or specific vaccines, such as the human papillomavirus vaccine. These groups meet as often as biweekly by teleconference. When developing recommendations concerning vaccination, the ACIP considers the vaccine-preventable disease burden, the effectiveness and safety of vaccines for various demographic groups, and cost-effectiveness. Its recommendations become effective when they are published in the CDC's *Morbidity and Mortality Weekly Report.*

The CDC accepts most ACIP recommendations (Smith 2008). The recommendation development process engages CDC staff throughout, most importantly as participants in workgroups and through comment on proposed recommendations at the public hearings. As assessed by the assistant to the CDC director of Immunization Policy, although "the committee can and does make its own independent recommendations, the process informs the committee about CDC staff views which they then take into account and informs CDC staff of other people's views which the CDC staff take into account. This process is very different from other advisory committee processes and, in large part, accounts for the high rate of CDC acceptance of ACIP recommendations" (Smith 2008).

The ACIP shares with private rulemaking the authority to determine the content of at least one type of rule. Indeed, the delegation is de jure rather than de facto. Although it differs from private rulemaking in that its members are appointed by government rather than selected by stakeholders, it explicitly involves stakeholders in the development process through the liaison representatives.

UK National Institute for Health and Clinical Excellence

Great care must be taken in drawing comparative public policy lessons (Marmor, Freeman, and Okma 2005). Differences in political institutions may make lessons drawn from one country irrelevant or worse when applied in another country. Drawing lessons about medical governance for the United States from other industrialized countries requires special caution because of fundamental differences in health care systems. Nonetheless, the National Institute for Health and Clinical Excellence (NICE) in the United Kingdom warrants consideration for a number of reasons, including its broad mission to advise on the clinical efficacy and cost-effectiveness of health technologies in England and Wales and the favorable international attention it has received (Schlander 2007).

Originally established as the National Institute for Clinical Excellence in 1999, NICE is a special health authority within the National Health Service funded by the government but with its own board of directors. The directors, appointed by an independent appointments commission, select the NICE executives—observers have compared the independence of NICE with that of the U.S. Federal Reserve Board (Pearson and Rawlins 2005). Nice is organized into three centers: the Centre for Public Health Excellence, which develops guidelines relevant to the promotion of good health and the prevention of ill health; the Centre for Clinical Practice, which develops guidelines for the treatment of specific diseases; and the Centre for Health Technology Evaluation, which assesses new and existing drugs, medical devices, diagnostic techniques, surgical procedures, and other treatments. NICE guidelines are effectively standards rather than rules in the American use of the terms. However, since 2002 the technology appraisals developed by the Centre for Health Technology Evaluation have been rules in that National Health Service Organizations in England and Wales are required to make available recommended medicines and treatments within three months.

NICE organizes independent advisory bodies consisting of researchers, medical practitioners, and patient advocates. The advisory committees conduct systematic reviews of all evidence relevant to clinical and economic assessment. Advisory committees work transparently, with stakeholder involvement throughout the assessment process. Indeed, transparency is a hallmark of NICE, which makes available all the data used by committees in reaching conclusions except for the details of certain proprietary information provided by manufacturers.

NICE is not without critics. For example, Michael Schlander provides a detailed critique of the appraisal process as it was applied to treatments for attention-deficit and hyperactivity disorder, finding weaknesses with respect to the scope of the appraisal, the decisions made regarding the included data, assumptions about treatment compliance, synthesis of data across studies, the economic modeling, and the handling of appeals (2007). Nonetheless, NICE appears to have been successful in establishing its credibility as a rigorous and independent organization. For example, the NICE proposal to eliminate funding for drugs to treat Alzheimer disease because they were not cost-effective elicited strong negative reactions in the media as an attack on the elderly. Nonetheless, the prime minister defended the independence of NICE on the floor of the House of Commons without opposition (Pearson and Rawlins 2005, 2622). NICE's technology appraisals are influential by virtue of their status as rules. The impact of its clinical guidance is less clear, however. A study of adherence to twelve of the earliest NICE guidelines found considerable variance across the acute, primary, and mental health trusts that are responsible for delivering medical care (Sheldon et al. 2004).

NICE is the most prominent institution that by explicit design routinely integrates cost-effectiveness analysis into its policy decisions. Its appraisal committees to the greatest extent possible assess the value of medical technologies in terms of their cost per quality-adjusted life year. NICE has not set a threshold value for this ratio, however, but instead considers it as a component of the appraisal. Rather than setting a threshold, which would effectively determine the budget of the National Health Service, NICE can be thought of as "seeking to identify the optimal threshold that lies somewhere between the least cost-effective technology currently in use and the most cost-effective technology not yet available routinely" (Culyer et al. 2007, 56).

In practice, concerns have been raised that the emphasis placed in appraisals on the quality of evidence tends to favor clinical findings, which often come from random trials, over economic evidence, which tends to include data from various sources and cannot avoid employing a variety of assumptions (Wailoo et al. 2004). Nonetheless, NICE is a rare example, joined only by the drug formularies of some countries and Canadian provinces, of the explicit and systematic integration of clinical and economic evidence in policy-making.

Although NICE neither is governed by stakeholders nor formally relies on them in its decision making, it has several other attributes of private rulemaking. Most important, it enjoys considerable independence from the National Health Service (and other ministries) and it produces rules, its technology appraisals, that have substantial consequences for the allocation of resources. It also conducts its appraisals with a high degree of transparency that facilitates extensive stakeholder participation.

Conclusion

Although neither unregulated markets nor isolated bureaus are viable alternatives for medical governance, a wide range of collaborative arrangements between government agencies and advisory bodies are possible. Public rulemaking supported by advisory committees is only one such arrangement. A very different arrangement is private rulemaking through an organization of stakeholders. The next five chapters consider one private rulemaker, the Organ Procurement and Transplantation Network, in considerable detail to assess the claims set out about the potential technical efficiency of private rulemaking and the opportunities and risks its poses.

Ideally, one would want to assess public versus private rulemaking by making empirical comparisons of the sort Cheit makes between public and private standard-setting (1990). Unfortunately, we do not have multiple cases of private rulemaking as a form of medical governance to study. Further, for the case that is available, we do not have directly parallel governance through public rulemaking as a basis for comparison. One of the reasons for reviewing public rulemaking in considerable depth is to provide a counterfactual against which to compare the case of private rulemaking that we do assess. The underlying assumption is that public rulemaking applied to organ transplantation would operate like public rulemaking in other contexts. Or, as John Gerring puts it: "One knows what blue is without going in search of blue cases" (2004, 347).

3

The Organ Procurement
and Transplantation Network

Federal transplantation policy in the United States evolved to produce the Organ
Procurement and Transplantation Network (OPTN) primarily in response to developments concerning two solid organs: kidneys and livers. Kidney transplantation initially
became important because it is a lower-cost alternative to dialysis for end-stage renal disease (ESRD) that offers higher quality of life and greater longevity. Liver transplantation
initially became important because of the publicity created by desperate parents seeking
organ donations and financial support for transplantations needed to save the lives of
those children. Although hearts, pancreases, intestines, and lungs are now commonly
transplanted, livers and kidneys continue to be the primary focal points for debates about
the allocation of transplant organs.

Experimental kidney transplantation had begun in 1951, but the first real success
came in 1954 with a case involving an isograft, or transplant between identical twins
(Tilney 2003). With the introduction of immunosuppressive drugs, which provided a way
of countering organ rejection, and with the development of the artificial kidney, which
allowed patients with kidney failure to be kept alive through dialysis while they waited for
transplant operations, kidney transplants between other-than identical twins, or allografts,
became common during the 1960s.

The powerful immunosuppressant cyclosporine, which began clinical trials in the
United States in 1980, had significant impacts on transplantation generally. The most
immediate was in reversing the generally disappointing results of liver transplants. Pediatric liver transplantation came to public attention dramatically in 1982 with the ultimately successful efforts of the parents of eleven-month-old Jamie Fiske to secure a liver
donation (Rettig 1989, 199). President Ronald Reagan, House Speaker Thomas O'Neill,
and newscaster Dan Rather all used their influence and media access on behalf of particular families seeking donors or financial support for pediatric liver transplants. A presidential aid, who helped pressure a number of states to cover the costs of liver transplants
under Medicaid, candidly remarked when interviewed for a weekly newspaper article:
"Sure, it's politics of the first order. It's whoever can get to the White House, whoever can
use the media" (Wehr 1984, 455). As one senator said at the time, "Are you going to have
every individual who needs an organ have to get next to the president?" (453).

Cooperation in Voluntary Networks

The allocation of cadaveric organs was not nearly as haphazard as media coverage suggested, however. Transplant centers were linked in informal networks that facilitated organ sharing. In economic terms, organs are heterogeneous goods. They differ in many ways relevant to transplantation: size, blood type, antigenicity, and overall quality. Consequently, it was not always possible for transplant centers to use all the cadaveric organs they recovered so that sharing among centers was mutually beneficial.

During the 1960s, transplant surgeons established kidney sharing networks based in Boston, Los Angeles, and Richmond (Dennis 1995, 101–2). Because cadavers usually provide two kidneys, the general practice for network members was to use one kidney locally, if possible, and to make the other available to the network. To ensure an equitable distribution of kidneys across transplant centers, the sharing procedures usually involved some sort of payback provisions that either required centers receiving a shared kidney to compensate the originating center with a kidney that would otherwise be locally used or gave priority in allocation to patients at centers that were net exporters of kidneys.

The federal government played a role in strengthening the informal networks as part of a general strategy to promote kidney transplantation. In the 1960s kidney transplantation became generally recognized as a medically desirable and cost-effective alternative to dialysis. In 1969, the Public Health Service gave contracts to seven hospitals to establish organizations to procure cadaveric kidney donations as well as a contract to UCLA to operate a computer system for matching donors and patients in the western states (Rettig 1989, 194). The Social Security Act Amendments of 1972 (Public Law 92-603) extended Medicare coverage for either dialysis or transplantation to patients with chronic renal disease through the ESRD program. Seeking to reduce the costs of the ESRD program by encouraging more kidney transplants, amendments to the Social Security Act in 1978 (Public Law 95-292) further increased financial accessibility by extending coverage for immunosuppressive drugs following transplants from one to three years. Further, in 1976, the Centers for Disease Control and Prevention initiated programs to promote organ donation and improve acquisition (Rettig 1989, 195).

Although the federal role in transplantation arose primarily through its interest in kidney transplantation, transplant surgeons also sought to involve the federal government in nonrenal—mainly liver and heart—transplantation as a route to obtaining private insurance coverage. As long as Medicare classified nonrenal transplantation as experimental, many private insurers would not provide coverage. An important event in this process was a consensus development conference on liver transplantation sponsored by the National Institutes of Health in 1983 at the urging of several members of Congress and Surgeon General Charles Everett Koop, who was particularly interested in promoting pediatric liver transplantation (Markle and Chubin 1987). Based on the recognition of liver transplantation by the conference as a promising treatment for many forms of liver disease, Medicare rules were changed the following year to pay for liver transplants for children who qualified for Medicare, an empty set. Jeffrey Prottas noted the catch-22 nature of this change: "The federal government agreed to pay for liver transplantation on the understanding that it would not have to do so" (1994, 128). More important for liver transplantation, its new status in Medicare opened the door for greater coverage by private insurance. Efforts by transplant surgeons eventually also led to Medicare coverage of heart transplants. A perhaps unintended consequence of these efforts, however, was greater federal involvement.

An existing network, the South-Eastern Regional Organ Procurement Program (SEOPP), sponsored by the Medical College of Virginia, was one of seven organizations originally funded by the Public Health Service in 1969 (Rettig 1989). Its membership initially consisted of eight transplant centers in four states and the District of Columbia (Pierce and McDonald 1996). The SEOPP introduced a computerized kidney matching system shortly after its creation. By 1975 its membership had expanded to eighteen transplant centers and it incorporated as the South-Eastern Organ Procurement Foundation. In response to requests from nonmembers to have their patients listed in the matching system, the foundation established the United Network for Organ Sharing (UNOS) in 1977 to facilitate nationwide matching of donated organs and patients. In 1982 the foundation and UNOS set up the Kidney Center, later called the Organ Center, to provide around-the-clock capacity to use the computer matching system to locate recipients for available organs. It also attempted to locate organs for the most critically ill patients through a classification system called UNOS/STAT. Thus, by 1983, UNOS was the only organization operating a nationwide system to support organ sharing (Denny 1983, 26).

Both its success in assuming a national role and its anticipation of federal legislation then under discussion led to the incorporation of UNOS as a nonprofit, voluntary membership organization in 1984. Its goals as outlined in its articles of incorporation were to establish a national organ procurement and transplantation network; improve the effectiveness of organ procurement, distribution, and transplantation systems; develop, implement, and maintain quality assurance activities; and systematically gather, analyze, and publish data related to transplantation (Pierce and McDonald 1996, 2). At its inception, UNOS was governed by a board of directors consisting of one representative from each member organization.

Several factors contributed to the rise of a private organization as a network administrative organization (NAO) to facilitate the national sharing of organs. First, from a functional perspective, networks allowed transplant centers to gain from what economists call a network externality. By voluntarily joining forces to expand the pools of donors and patients, the centers were able to increase the effective use of the heterogeneous organs available so that on average all were better off in terms of finding appropriate organs for their patients. The network externality was strong enough to result in the eventual emergence of a single national network. If organs were homogenous by type (for example, all kidneys were interchangeable), then there would be no network externality and one would not expect voluntary networks to arise.

Second, from a sociological perspective, the networks were formed by surgeons who shared professional norms and relationships that facilitated cooperation. Although saving lives at one's center was most rewarding, contributing to saving lives anywhere in the network was consistent with medial professionalism. Transplant surgeons also often knew each other personally by virtue of their mutual participation in professional societies and often through their shared experiences training at major transplant centers. Thus participants brought common values and often personal trust to the networks.

Third, the federal government took a number of steps that indirectly and directly promoted the creation or strengthening of networks. Most important, the coverage of ESRD costs for patients of any age under Medicare greatly expanded the number of patients for whom a kidney transplant was financially feasible. More directly, the support of local networks to increase the procuring and sharing of organs and the establishment of computer systems for matching donors and patients by the Public Health Service reinforced and legitimized the developing networks.

Fourth, the emergence of UNOS as an NAO is consistent with the predictions of Keith Provan and Patrick Kenis concerning network governance (2008). In particular, it follows their predictions that an NAO will emerge when the need for network-level competencies is high, levels of trust and consensus on network-level goals are moderately high, and the number of participants is moderate to large. UNOS also helped deal with the problem of external legitimacy facing transplant centers, convincing the public that the allocation of scarce organs was fair, or at least based on medical considerations, and the network problem of internal legitimacy, convincing transplant centers that they were receiving their fair shares from participation in the network, the sort of important balancing that Proven and Kenis see NAOs as providing.

Network Formalization:
The National Organ Transplant Act

Organ transplantation received increasing levels of newspaper and television coverage during the early 1980s (Rettig 1989, 208). In 1983, Rep. Albert Gore (D–TN), chairman of the Subcommittee on Investigations and Oversight of the House Committee on Science and Technology, held hearings that focused on children who received or were seeking liver transplants. The following year he worked with several members of Congress, including Rep. Henry Waxman (D–CA) and Sen. Orrin Hatch (R–UT) and Sen. Edward Kennedy (D–MA), to craft legislation to create a formal, but privately administered network, the Organ Procurement and Transplantation Network, to encourage more effective procurement of cadaveric organs and to coordinate their allocation. Although the Reagan administration initially opposed the creation of a national network to replace voluntary efforts, the passage of the Senate version, S. 2048, by voice vote, and the overwhelming support (396 to 6) for the House version of the bill, H.R. 5580, encouraged President Reagan to sign the National Organ Transplant Act (Public Law 98-507) into law on October 19, 1984.

The act called for the secretary of the Department of Health and Human Services (HHS) to contract with a not-for-profit organization to establish and operate the OPTN, which would, among other responsibilities, maintain a national list of patients awaiting transplants to facilitate matching them with donated organs on the basis of medical criteria. Title I of the act established a twenty-one-member Task Force on Organ Transplantation to prepare a report with recommendations concerning the operation of the OPTN. The act also prohibited commerce in organs by making it unlawful for any person knowingly to "acquire, receive, or otherwise transfer any human organ for valuable consideration for use in human transplantation if the transfer affects interstate commerce" (Title III, Sec. 101a).

The report recommended that "each donated organ be considered a national resource to be used for the public good" and that the selection of patients for inclusion on waiting lists and the allocation of organs to them "be based on medical criteria that are publicly stated and fairly applied" (Task Force on Organ Transplantation 1986, 9). Medical criteria should "take into account both need and probability of success" (10). The report strongly endorsed the prohibition against the commercialization of organs (10), but rejected the creation of a national list of donors. It argued instead for obtaining consent from next-of-kin, so as to give them the opportunity for an altruistic act, an approach that, as discussed in chapter 4, has had significant implications for organ procurement from those who pledged them while alive (Blumstein 1989, 27–28). In what turned out to involve the "most vigorous and divisive debates" among Task Force members (Childress 1989, 105), it responded to concerns prompted by reports that some centers provided transplants to large numbers of wealthy foreign patients by recommending that no more than 10 percent of cadaveric kidneys be allocated to nonimmigrant aliens at any transplant center and that extrarenal (other than the kidney) organs not be offered to nonimmigrant aliens unless no other suitable recipient could be found (Task Force on Organ Transplantation 1986, 10). Among the other recommendations was a call to establish a board to advise the secretary of HHS on organ transplantation policy (13).

The status of the OPTN was strengthened somewhat in the Omnibus Reconciliation Act of 1986 (Public Law 99-509), which required all hospitals performing organ transplants to be members of the OPTN and to abide by its rules to receive payments under Medicare and Medicaid. It was further strengthened by Title IV of the Omnibus Health Amendments of 1988 (Public Law 100-607), which required the OPTN to "establish membership criteria and medical criteria for allocating organs and provide to members of the public an opportunity to comment with respect to such criteria" (Sec. 403a). Subsequently, HHS interpreted the laws to require any rules to be approved by the secretary before they are binding on OPTN members (1989), and clarified the circumstances of approval in an extended and controversial rulemaking beginning in 1994 and finalized in 2000 that is discussed in chapter 5 (2000). Even if the OPTN had retained unilateral authority to expel members, doing so would be so draconian, because the threat of loss of all Medicare and Medicaid participation would force hospitals to shut down expelled transplant programs completely, that it would probably not have been a credible threat. Although the secretary must approve all OPTN rules before they become enforceable as federal rules, the OPTN can discipline members who fail to comply by designating them as not in good standing. Because HHS has yet to accept formally any substantive OPTN rules through a federal rulemaking, the OPTN effectively retains responsibility for developing the content of the rules themselves. As Prottas summarized it, "public policy makers may not choose to set the nation's rules for organ allocation directly, but they can do so" (1994, 148).

The contract for administering the OPTN and the Scientific Registry of Transplant Recipients (SRTR), a data base for assessing transplant results, was awarded in 1986 to UNOS. Since then UNOS has continued to secure contracts for administration of the OPTN, though in 2000 it lost the contract for administering the SRTR to the University Renal Research and Education Association, now the Arbor Research Collective for Health, a nonprofit organization based in Ann Arbor, Michigan.

Overview of the OPTN and Its Governance

The OPTN is an example of private rulemaking: although ultimate responsibility for mandatory rules lies de jure with the HHS secretary, stakeholders de facto design the content of the rules and oversee their implementation. The mission of the OPTN is set out in article II of its charter (as revised in 2004):

> The primary purposes of the OPTN are to operate and monitor an equitable system for allocating organs donated for transplantation; maintain a waiting list of potential recipients; match potential recipients with organ donors according to established medical criteria for allocation of organs and, to the extent feasible, for listing and de-listing transplant patients; facilitate the efficient, effective placement of organs for transplantation; and increase organ donation. To accomplish these purposes, the OPTN:
>
> (a) Establishes, maintains, and monitors compliance with voluntary and mandatory membership criteria/policies and procedures for institutions and interested parties and training and experience criteria as consistent with Federal regulations for primary personnel at transplant programs. Policies may become mandatory through a process involving consideration and recommendation as a mandatory policy by the OPTN and official adoption by the Secretary of the Department of Health and Human Services (HHS) of the policy as mandatory.
>
> (b) Establishes, maintains, and monitors compliance with voluntary and mandatory criteria/policies and procedures for the safe and efficient acquisition and transportation of donor organs and for the allocation and distribution of these organs equitably among transplant patients, consistent with Federal law and regulations. Policies may become mandatory through a process involving consideration and recommendation as a mandatory policy by the OPTN and official adoption by the Secretary of HHS of the policy as mandatory.
>
> (c) Collects, analyzes, and publishes data on pre-transplant and post-transplant events to advance the fields of organ transplantation, organ procurement, organ preservation, and immunogenetics. (http://optn.transplant.hrsa.gov/policiesAndBylaws/)

Funding for operation of the OPTN comes from two sources. The larger is a registration fee paid by transplant centers when they place a patient on the transplant list. The current fee is $502 per registration. In fiscal year 2007 (October 1, 2007 through September 30, 2008) 50,629 registrations yielded more than $25 million in revenue. The federal government provides $2 million annually as part of the contract with UNOS for administration of the network. Together, these sources funded a budget of $26.7 million in fiscal year 2007.

The OPTN has six types of voting members: transplant centers, organ procurement organizations, histocompatibility laboratories, professional and medical organizations, scientific organizations, voluntary health organizations, and general public members. The transplant centers, procurement organizations, and laboratories must be members in order to participate in transplantation involving federal funding. The professional and voluntary organizations join because transplantation is relevant to their missions. Members from the general public have expertise or interests, typically based on firsthand experience, relevant to transplantation.

Currently 254 transplant centers located in hospitals are OPTN members. Almost all of the centers, 245, transplant kidneys. In terms of the other solid organs, 145 centers transplant pancreases, 126 transplant livers, 132 are authorized to transplant hearts (but only 126 are currently active), 66 transplant lungs, and 45 transplant intestines.

The territory of the United States is divided into fifty-eight geographic areas called donation service areas (DSAs). In each DSA an organ procurement organization (OPO) has responsibility for procuring deceased-donor organs. Each OPO has a monopoly over procuring organs from cadavers in hospitals within its geographic area. Fifty of the OPOs are independent organizations that harvest cadaveric organs from multiple hospitals. The other eight are operated by transplant centers based in specific hospitals and do not hold independent membership in the OPTN.

Histocompatibility laboratories conduct tests of donors and patients in support of transplantation. Most prominently, they examine human leukocyte antigens, so-called tissue typing, to facilitate matching of donated kidneys and pancreases with suitable recipients. There are 154 histocompatibility laboratories, but 96 are operated by transplant centers and do not hold independent memberships in the OPTN.

Thirty professional and voluntary organizations are currently OPTN members. Not surprisingly, the twenty-one professional organizations include many directly concerned with transplantation, such as the American Society of Transplantation, the American Society of Transplant Surgeons, the Association of Organ Procurement Organizations, the American Society for Histocompatibility and Immunogenetics, the American Foundation for Donation and Transplantation, the Transplant Financial Coordinators Association, and the Society for Transplant Social Workers. Other professional organization members, such as the American Hospital Association and the National Association of Medical Examiners, have missions encompassing more than transplantation. Nine voluntary health organizations, including the National Kidney Foundation, the American Diabetes Association, and the Transplant Recipients International Organization, are also members. At the beginning of 2008, the OPTN had 392 member organizations. Seven people from the general public were also members by virtue of their service on the OPTN board of directors or committees. Total membership was thus 399.

The OPTN divides the Unites States into eleven regions relevant to the functioning of the OPTN in a number of ways. First, allocation rules for kidneys, pancreases, and intestines have a geographic hierarchy giving first priority to local patients (generally those registered in the transplant centers served by the OPO procuring the organ), next priority to patients at centers in the region, and finally to patients elsewhere in the United States. Livers are allocated initially at the regional level. (Hearts and lungs have their own geographic hierarchy based on distances.) Second, regions play a role in voting for members of the board of directors and other officers and they have representatives on the board of directors and all standing committees. Third, they play an administrative role in reviewing patient classifications for allocation of some organs, most prominently for livers. Fourth, regional meetings provide a forum for obtaining feedback and advisory votes on policy proposals.

The ultimate responsibility for setting OPTN policies lies with the board of directors, which includes all the members of board of directors of UNOS as well as nonvoting ex officio members from HHS. The board of directors has between thirty- four and forty-two elected members. Bylaws require that 50 percent of the directors be surgeons or physicians directly involved in transplantation and that at least 25 percent of the directors be organ donors, transplant candidates, or recipients, or their families recruited from the general public. Most directors serve two-year terms, but the general public directors and those from voluntary health organizations serve three-year terms.

Voting within the OPTN for directors, officers, and regional representatives depends on the class of membership. Each hospital (transplant center) has one voting representative, as does each independent OPO. Histocompatibility laboratories have thirty-three voting representatives, two per region and eleven elected at large for two-year terms. Professional organizations have twenty-four, elected at large for two-year terms. Voluntary organizations have twelve, with at least one from each region, if possible, elected for two-year terms. Finally, general public members also have twelve, one from each region and the twelfth selected by the eleven for a two-year term. Voting members in each region elect a councilor and an associate councilor, who both generally serve as members of the board of directors. The remaining vacancies on the board of directors are filled through election at the annual membership meeting.

The principal officers of the OPTN include the president and vice president, who serve one-year terms, and the vice president for patient and donor affairs, secretary, and treasurer, who serve two-year terms. A salaried executive director, who serves at the pleasure of the board of directors, oversees the UNOS staff, who support day-to-day operations of the OPTN, including the work of the committees.

Although the board of directors makes final decisions on OPTN policies, the bulk of the substantive work is done by standing committees that include regional and general public representatives as well as relevant experts drawn from institutional members. The committees are organized by organ, cross-cutting issues, and administration. The current organ-specific committees are kidney transplantation, liver and intestinal organ transplantation, pancreas transplantation, and thoracic organ transplantation (hearts and lungs). The cross-cutting committees are ethics, living donor, minority affairs, histocompatibility, OPO, organ availability, patient affairs, and pediatric transplantation. The two most important administrative committees are membership and professional standards and policy oversight.

The committees make extensive use of studies based on data from the SRTR as well as on the relevant tacit knowledge of their members, most of whom are active practitioners. In addition to including general public representatives as voting members on both committees and the board of directors, participation comes in several other forms. Committees often seek comments and advisory votes from regions and their proposals are routinely reviewed by other committees. In some cases, committees have held public meetings to obtain input relevant to major policy issues. For example, in February 2007

Table 3–1   Summary of Governance Arrangements for Organ Transplantation

	OPTN	SRTR
Administrator	United Network for Organ Sharing	Arbor Research Collective for Health
Funding (FY 2007)	federal contract, $2 million listing fees, $25 million	federal contract, $3.8 million
Independent organizational members	254 transplant centers 50 organ procurement organizations 58 histocompatability laboratories 30 professional and voluntary organizations	—
Decision making	board of directors, 34 to 42 voting members	technical advisory committee, 8 to 10 voting members

the Kidney Committee held a public forum with more than five hundred participants to discuss proposals for major revisions of kidney allocation rules. The board of directors routinely initiates public comment periods on proposed policy changes.

In summary, the OPTN organizational structure facilitates the consideration of both scientific information based on the comprehensive collection of data on transplantation and the tacit knowledge of practitioners, patients, and others with an interest in transplantation. Policy changes move forward based on voting within committees and finally by voting within the board of directors. This relatively transparent policymaking process produces continuous incremental change in policy. Table 3–1 summarizes the governance of the OPTN and its sister institution, the SRTR.

Standardization versus Experimentation in Allocation Rules

In a country as large and diverse as the United States, some variation in national policy may be desirable, both to fit policy better to local circumstances and to provide a basis for policy experimentation. Waivers, which allow states to deviate from federal policy, have been widely used in the Medicaid program to encourage experimentation with community-based long-term care (Miller, Ramsland, and Harrington 1999), service delivery, financing, and coverage options (Schneider 1997). The use of waivers may have played a role in preserving Medicaid as an entitlement against efforts to convert it to a block grant program (Thompson and Burke 2007). Waivers were also used extensively in the Aid to Families with Dependent Children program before welfare reform (Ziliak et al. 2000). From its beginning, the OPTN has allowed waivers, called variances, that permit deviations from national policy. Initially, many of these variances were granted to permit OPOs to continue policies already in place before the OPTN was established. Over time, however, variances have become mainly mechanisms for facilitating policy experiments.

Variances have two primary forms: alternative allocation units and alternative allocation rules. Each OPO maintains a list of all patients locally eligible for transplants. OPOs that are geographically large or consist of noncontiguous areas may seek to divide into alternative local units with separate patient lists. OPOs in contiguous and geographically compact areas may seek to create an alternative allocation unit that allows them to merge their waiting lists, effectively moving the primary basis of allocation from the local to the regional level. OPOs or regions wishing to apply alternative rules for allocating a particular organ may obtain variances that allow them to do so. Most variances are initiated by OPOs, though in several instances the OPTN has approved a committee-sponsored variance intended to recruit OPOs into particular experiments.

The use of variances for facilitating policy experiments got off to a shaky start. A U.S. General Accounting Office report completed in 1993 found that a quarter of OPOs were not using comprehensive allocation lists and that OPOs with variances were generally not providing data to demonstrate that the variances were meeting their intended goals. In response, the OPTN adopted a policy that defined the local unit for organ allocation to be the OPO. In addition, it adopted new procedures for approving variances to national allocation rules and assessing their impacts. A follow-up report in 1995 found that the OPTN had been successful in making the OPO the basic local unit for allocation but still fell short in terms of its evaluation of variances. Of the twenty-two variances in allocation rules then in effect, only one OPO had submitted all the requested reports and only one provided data that the Government Accounting Office analysts judged as adequate for assessing whether the variance was achieving its goals.

Over time, the OPTN increased the reporting requirements to provide a much stronger basis for evaluating the impacts of variances. Currently, variances are granted initially for three years, with annual reporting requirements. During this period, the variance holder must demonstrate that the variance is meeting its goals. In the case of committee-sponsored variances, the purpose is expressly experimental. Specific time limits are set and the sponsoring committee has responsibility for conducting the evaluation of the variance. As discussed in chapters 5 and 6, variances have produced information that has contributed to changes in allocation policy for both livers and kidneys.

Quality Control, Compliance, and Enforcement

The OPTN has responsibility for establishing requirements for membership. These requirements largely involve the types and professional training and experience of personnel. For example, each transplant center must have a primary surgeon, primary physician, clinical transplant coordinator, and financial coordinator. To establish a new transplant program, a hospital must document that it meets the requirements for membership. The documentation undergoes medical peer review by the Membership and Professional Standards Committee (MPSC), which makes a recommendation for granting membership to the board of directors.

The distinction between federal rules, which have legal authority, and OPTN rules, which have only intraorganizational authority, limit the sanctions that the OPTN can apply to members who do not comply with policies and bylaws. HHS has taken a restrained approach to making OPTN policies federal rules. None of the organ allocation rules have been made mandatory. Indeed, the only OPTN policies issued as federal regulations have been related to data and event reporting requirements. The OPTN does not have the legal basis for removal of designated status of a transplant program that failed to provide required data or, say, for a transplant program that failed to follow liver allocation rules. If the OPTN wishes to terminate a transplant hospital's participation in Medicare or Medicaid, which would effectively shut it down, because it has not complied with allocation rules, it can only recommend this action to HHS. In 2006, for the first time, the OPTN recommended that the designated transplant program status for two transplant programs be removed. The secretary accepted these recommendations.

The OPTN can impose costs of various sorts on a noncomplying organizational member by designating it as on probation or, more drastically, as a member not in good standing. Probation can involve one or more of the following interventions: required preparation of a corrective plan to meet specifications set by the MPSC, adherence to the plan, and documentation of its execution; unscheduled on-site surveys of compliance by UNOS staff at the expense of the member; and required submission of specific data, reports, and other evidence to document compliance. Being a member not in good standing can result in any of the interventions available for probation, as well as suspension of participation in OPTN governance (loss of voting rights and loss of the opportunity for personnel associated with the member organization to serve on committees or hold office) and notification of the adverse action to OPTN members, the general public, the relevant health official in the member's state, and the member's patients. Thus, short of suspension or withdrawal of membership, failure to comply with OPTN rules puts the member at risk for increased compliance costs, ostracism from the network, and a tarnished reputation for its sponsoring hospital as well as for its professional staff.

The MPSC conducts both routine reviews of transplant programs that meet specific screening criteria as well as investigations in response to complaints or specific incidents brought to its attention. If either of these processes leads the MPSC to recommend that the board of directors take an adverse action (probation, designation as member not in good standing, or request for suspension of membership rights), then due process procedures become available to the member. Members may dispute adverse actions through the following sequence of appeals: provision of new information to the MPSC; an interview with the MPSC; a formal hearing before the MPSC; a formal hearing before the board of directors; and, finally, a written appeal to the HHS secretary.

In each of the cases involving designation of a member as not in good standing, the member pursued a reversal as far as through the formal hearing before the board of directors. In one case, a routine site visit and audit of patient data by UNOS staff discovered that St. Vincent Medical Center had accepted a liver for an unavailable patient but actually transplanted it into another patient rather than releasing it for allocation to the next person on the waiting list. Further, the transplant program falsely reported to the OPTN that it had transplanted the liver into the original patient, who was therefore removed from the list and subsequently died waiting for a transplant. Although St. Vincent pledged its full commitment to a corrective plan, the OPTN president, Francis Delmonico, stated that "the MPSC and the OPTN/UNOS Board of Directors also believe that the Member Not in Good Standing sanction is appropriate to call attention to the failure of the institutional control which allowed these serious violations to occur and be covered up for an extended period. Therefore, the Board's action should send a very clear message to the transplant community, and to the general public, that our responsibilities, as stewards of the gift of donated organs, cannot be compromised" (UNOS 2006a, 1).

The second case involved Kaiser Permanente. It established a kidney transplant program and stopped paying for transplants at other centers for its health network subscribers with end-stage renal disease living in northern California, after which the number of transplants received by its subscribers declined significantly. Although Kaiser Permanente agreed to transfer its patients to other transplant centers and then close its kidney transplant program, the OPTN president, Sue McDiarmid, argued that "the designation of Member Not in Good Standing is warranted to note the institution's lapses that effectively denied patient access to kidney transplantation and threatened safety for patients on the waiting list" (UNOS 2006b, 1).

Adverse actions are rare—indeed, the St. Vincent and Kaiser Permanente cases are the only ones resulting in the member-not-in-good-standing designation. Much more frequently, the MPSC conducts routine reviews of transplant programs for whom one-year patient survival rates suggest a potential quality or compliance problem. From 1999 through 2005, the MPSC conducted 261 reviews of transplant programs with potential quality problems detected from a report card prepared by the SRTR (OPTN/SRTR 2005, VIII-16).

An organizational report card can be defined as "a regular effort by an organization to collect data on two or more *other organizations*, transform the data into information relevant to assessing performance, and transmit the information to some audience external to the organizations themselves" (Gormley and Weimer 1999, 3). The SRTR bases its report cards on the data it collects on transplant patients. It transforms these data into information about the relative performance of transplant programs by calculating risk-adjusted mortality rates for each center. The risk-adjustment process involves using the national data to estimate statistical models relating patient and donor characteristics to the probability of survival after various periods of time. Prediction for individual patients permits comparisons of the expected and observed rates for transplant programs. Descriptive and risk-adjusted outcome measures for each transplant program, along with regional and national figures for ease of comparison, are made available to the public, including prospective transplant patients, online (www.ustransplant.org/csr/current/csrDefault.aspx).

In addition to facilitating bottom-up pressure for quality improvement by providing information to transplant consumers, the report card also facilitates top-down monitoring by the MPSC and, more recently, by HHS. On a quarterly basis, the SRTR prepares an updated list of transplant programs by organ that presents expected and observed one-year death, graft failure, and survival rates for two successive transplant cohorts, but without the transplant center's name or location identified. Currently, larger programs (more than ten transplants per cohort) that meet three criteria for two successive cohorts of patients are screened by the MPSC for review: the ratio of observed to expected one-year deaths is greater than 1.5, the difference between the number of observed and expected one-year deaths is greater than 3, and this difference is statistically significant in a one-sided test at the 5 percent level. About 7 to 10 percent of programs meet the three criteria (OPTN/ SRTR 2005, VIII-12). Because smaller programs (ten or fewer transplants per cohort) rarely meet these criteria, they are subjected to a separate annual review if they experience one or more deaths.

The MPSC requests audit reports from all screened transplant programs. The reports verify patient data, discuss the circumstances of each death and graft failure, and allow centers to indicate any unique clinical factors that may be relevant to the outcomes. Based on the reports, the MPSC makes a decision about whether to release the program from review or follow-up with a site visit. If it makes specific recommendations, it subsequently monitors compliance. Failure to implement the recommendations would generally result in an adverse action.

In 2007 the Centers for Medicare and Medicaid Services (CMS) began its own monitoring of the quality of transplant centers based on its authority to oversee facilities participating in Medicare. Its general approach relies primarily on data already being collected and reports already being produced by the SRTR and supplementation of the oversight already being done by the OPTN. For example, in determining eligibility for Medicare participation, the CMS begins its quality assessment using the same screening criteria the MPSC uses. In responding to comments received in response to the proposed rule, the CMS justified its additional oversight as follows:

> The OPTN generally takes a collegial approach and assists centers in improving their performance, while we generally take a regulatory approach which sometimes may lead to termination of the Medicare agreement with providers. However, compliance with the OPTN's policies will facilitate transplant centers' compliance with the requirements of this final rule. Therefore, the OPTN will continue to play a consultative role with transplant centers to assist them in complying with Medicare requirements. We believe the collegial relationship between the OPTN and the transplant centers may be enhanced and strengthened rather than compromised. (HHS 2007b, 15209)

In light of the controversy between HHS and UNOS during the late 1990s, which is discussed in chapter 5, it is interesting to note the CMS response to a comment raising concerns about codifying OPTN policies:

> The requirements in this final rule are intended to be broadly applicable to transplant centers over a long period of time. OPTN policies or elements of OPTN policies that we have included in this final rule conform to this intent. We understand that many OPTN policies, particularly organ allocation, transplant surgeon and transplant physician credentials, and criteria for listing and de-listing transplant candidates are subject to rapid changes as transplant medicine advances. Therefore, we did not include such policies in this final rule. (HHS 2007b, 15209)

These excerpts illustrate two important claims about distinctions between private and public rulemaking made in chapter 2. First, private rulemaking is generally more cooperative and less adversarial. Second, private rulemaking tends to be more flexible in incorporating new information into rules.

Conclusion

The OPTN, both a network administrative organization and a de facto private rulemaker, evolved from an existing voluntary network of transplantation organizations. The network was professional, facilitating the sharing of knowledge in a rapidly evolving area of medicine, as well as functional, capturing a network externality through broader geographic sharing of heterogeneous organs. It was voluntary, enabling patients, and especially the desperate parents of pediatric patients, to use media access and political connections to seek and sometimes obtain organ donations, raising broad concerns among the public about the fairness of the organ transplantation system. Congress sought to create a governance system, consisting of the OPTN and the SRTR, that would engage those with expertise and interests in the development of medically valid and equitable rules for organ procurement and allocation. How well has the OPTN carried out its responsibilities? The next four chapters seek to answer this question.

4

———————◦◦◦◦———————

Expanding Organ Supply

Perhaps within our lifetimes stem cell technology will allow new organs to be grown to specification so that cadaveric and live organ donation will no longer be necessary. Until then, however, the scarcity of organs for transplantation creates what Guido Calabresi and Philip Bobbitt famously called a tragic choice (1978). Indeed, the choice inherent in organ transplantation is driven by constraints, unlike Calabresi and Bobbitt's canonical case of a limited supply of dialysis machines, that cannot be easily relaxed through additional investments of resources. Although the most controversial issues arising in the governance of organ transplantation have involved the allocation of cadaveric organs, policies related to the availability of transplant organs have remained important and the OPTN has played a role in shaping them.

The first successful transplants depended on kidneys from live donors, usually close relatives. The acceptance of the concept of brain death, however, opened the door for widespread use of cadaveric organs in transplantation, and it became ever more practical to go through the door with improvements in immosuppressive drugs and technology for preserving organs during their cold ischemic time. In addition to expanding the supply of organs for kidney transplantation, the availability of cadaveric organs permitted the transplantation of other organs for which donation from the living was not an option. Expansion of the supply of transplant organs has involved efforts to harvest more organs from donors who meet the standard criteria, the expansion of the cadaveric pool to donors beyond those who meet the standard donation criteria, and the facilitation of live donation through policies such as paired exchanges. The evolution of these organ supply policies has often involved controversy over the relative importance of the values of autonomy, altruism, and efficiency.

Basic Framework of Cadaveric Organ Donation

A small fraction of deaths create potentially useful organ donations: only eleven thousand to fourteen thousand of more than 2.3 million deaths annually in the United States meet the standard donation criteria (Sheehy et al. 2003). Standard donors suffer brain death in a hospital so that their heart can be kept beating after death until the organs are removed and properly stored, transported, and transplanted. These donors are generally sixty years

57

old or younger. Most commonly, they become potential donors following accidents or strokes.

Legal and Moral Foundations

The conversion of potential donors to actual donors depends on legal, social, and organizational factors. In the United States the legal status of cadaveric organ donation is determined primarily by states, all of which have adopted the Uniform Anatomical Gift Act. Originally formulated in 1968, the act was quickly adopted by all states. It was revised in 1987 and 2006 to make it more consistent with national organ policy, but not all states have adopted these revisions (National Conference of Commissioners on Uniform State Laws 2008). The basic act is consistent with the principles of self-ownership and informed consent: an organ belongs to the deceased and can be taken only with the consent of the deceased. Obviously, the deceased cannot give consent after death. They can give it before death, however, typically by indicating their desire to donate when they obtain drivers' licenses, write wills, or discuss their wishes with family members. Parents are assumed to know this intention for their unemancipated children. In the absence of an expressed desire to donate before death, the intentions of deceased adults are determined, in order of priority, by spouses, adult children, parents, adult siblings, adult grandchildren, grandparents, and other persons who exhibited special care or concern for the deceased or were appointed as guardians.

The act also guards against a potential conflict of interest: the physician who declares a person dead may not be directly involved in organ retrieval. Most donors receive intensive care before death. Because the transplant surgeons who extract organs almost never have any involvement in the medical care of donors, they do not have occasion to be involved directly in the determination of death. The provision thus primarily serves to reassure potential donors that no transplant-related conflict of interest will interfere with that determination.

In theory, the informed consent of the donor takes priority. In practice, however, donation usually does not occur unless family members consent to it. In an effort to honor better the wishes of the deceased to donate, most states have in recent years adopted first-person consent provisions that attempt to direct those involved in procuring organs to recover them even in the absence of family consent when potential donors have made their intentions to donate clear. Additionally, the most recent revision of the Uniform Anatomical Gift Act allows donation in the absence of expressed donor consent when one member of a priority class consents and none of the others object. So, for example, if there is no surviving spouse, donation may occur if only one of the adult children consents as long as no other adult children object. Most states that have adopted first-person consent laws have also created donor registries. These confidential databases provide lists of all state residents who have expressed the intention to donate. Because intentions are most often expressed when people obtain drivers' licenses or identification cards, most registries are administered either by, or in cooperation with, motor vehicle departments.

In contrast to informed consent, many countries rely on the principle of presumed consent for cadaveric organ donation. That is, instead of opting in, one must explicitly opt out if one does not wish to donate. Some countries, such as Austria and Brazil, use a strong form of implied consent, in which the families of deceased potential donors are not consulted. Other countries, such as Belgium and France, use a weaker form, in which family members are not sought out but may take the initiative to block a donation. In the United States, several states use a weak form of presumed consent for cornea donation, suggesting that presumed consent would be constitutionally viable (Wilcox 2003). However, switching to presumed consent for solid organs is unlikely, not only because it would raise objections from people who would view it as an inappropriate government interference in personal autonomy and property rights, but also because it would run counter to the ideology of altruism that has shaped the U.S. organ procurement system.

The social acceptance of cadaveric donation evolved as transplantation moved from an experimental to a clinical treatment. Kieran Healy draws parallels between supporting arguments made by the life insurance industry in the middle of the nineteenth century to gain acceptance of its product and those made by the emerging transplant industry over the last forty years to gain acceptance of organ donation (2006). Just as life insurance was touted as consolation in the anticipation of death, so too is organ donation, which enables one to anticipate saving lives and providing comfort to one's family as they grieve. Just as life insurance was presented as "a way to live on (and do good) after death" (Healy 2006, 33), so too is organ donation: the donor spiritually and physically lives on in the recipient. And just as life insurance came to be viewed as a moral act, so too has organ donation. Although issues related to the definition of death and the preservation of life prompted some religious leaders to raise concerns, the presumption of the morality of organ donation eventually became widespread as it gained acceptance from all major organized religions.

The moral foundation for organ donation is set firmly in altruism. The basic premise that organs should be viewed as a gift, freely given by donors, was already strongly held by physicians and medical ethicists before formulation of the Uniform Anatomical Gift Act. It was reinforced by the influential book *The Gift Relationship*, by Richard Titmuss (1971), which compares the altruistic blood donation system of the United Kingdom with the mixed commercial and altruistic blood donation system of the United States, arguing that the former not only promoted important social values, including altruism and sense of community, but also resulted in a higher quality and more efficient blood supply. Although not unchallenged (see, for example, Arrow 1972), the arguments Titmuss makes have been highly influential.

Embracing altruism as the fundamental value underlying donation has influenced public policy, and the resulting supply of organs, in two important ways. First, it supported the ban on the sale of organs that appeared in the National Organ Transplantation Act and it continues to provide a basis for opposing monetary incentives for donation. Second, it contributed to the notion promoted by the Task Force on Organ Transplantation that giving families the opportunity to make altruistic gifts was socially valuable.

In November 1983, while Representative Gore was holding hearings before the Sub-Committee on Investigations and Oversight of the Committee on Science and Technology on legislation to create the OPTN, a physician named H. Barry Jacobs announced plans to establish the International Kidney Exchange, which was intended to provide a market in which healthy people from around the world could sell one of their kidneys to those in need of a transplant (Healy 2006, 35). The proposal was denounced by such organizations as the National Kidney Foundation, the American Society of Transplantation Surgeons, and the Transplantation Society, as well as by a number of leading medical ethicists, who argued strongly for altruistic donation. It prompted Gore to add a provision prohibiting the sale of solid organs for transplantation in interstate commerce. This provision became part of the National Organ Transplant Act.

The Task Force on Organ Transplantation embraced altruism as the only appropriate basis for donation. The embrace was not just of the altruistic decision of the individual to donate before death but also of that by the family after death. As a basis for individual donation, altruism is fully consistent with autonomy. It is plausibly consistent with autonomy when the families of the deceased base their decision of whether to allow donation on their sincere assessment of the deceased's intentions. However, it directly conflicts with autonomy when families are allowed to override the expressed wishes of the deceased. Thus, giving families the opportunity to be altruistic by not procuring organs without their permission, even when the deceased has previously recorded a desire to donate, directly conflicts with the value of autonomy.

Embracing the promotion of altruism over autonomy had an important consequence for the path that organ procurement policy has followed. Congress had asked the Task Force to consider explicitly the desirability of creating a national donor list that would allow for the quick identification of the deceased who had previously expressed a wish to donate. Commenting on the decision of the Task Force not to recommend a national donor list, James Blumstein wrote: "The resistance to the establishment of a list of potential organ donors is another example of policy-inhibiting aspects of a set of hard ideological rules—there is no valuable consideration for allowing one's organs to be used after death for transplantation, an exclusive reliance on altruistic motivation for transplantable organ supply, and a total commitment to the purported benefits of communitarian expressions of solidarity through families' choosing to donate the organs of their next of kin at the time of death" (1989, 28).

Deferring to the wishes of the family even when they conflict with an individual's expressed wishes to donate can be defended on two grounds other than communitarian solidarity. First, the courts have historically recognized that families have a "quasi-property" right to the corpse (Childress 1989, 89). Consulting with families is consistent with this right. Second, from a practical perspective, it is not only difficult for procurement personnel to go against the wishes of families in the midst of their grief, it is also potentially damaging to public opinion, and hence the willingness of individuals to commit to donation before death and the willingness of families to permit donation in the absence of such commitment. Even in states that have adopted first-person consent laws, procurement personnel often continue to defer to the wishes of the family (Mesich-Brant and Grossback 2005).

Organizational Framework

Organ procurement organizations (OPOs) have local monopolies for procuring cadaveric organs within their donation service areas. Each of the fifty-eight OPOs receives payments from the Medicare program to cover the reasonable and documented costs of procuring organs, yielding what amounts to a price of procurement per organ, the standard acquisition charge, calculated as the total allowable costs divided by the number of organs procured and transplanted. The allowable costs include all pre-transplant services for recipients or potential recipients (services provided before admission to the hospital for the transplant operation) and all the costs associated with organ donors, whether alive or deceased (Abecassis 2006). (The actual transplant services not covered by private insurers are paid by Medicare through a diagnostic related group [DRG] prospective payment.) The standard acquisition charge varies by OPO and organ. For kidneys it ranges from about $16,000 to $32,000, depending on local cost circumstances, the degree of risk aversion the OPO accepts in claiming reasonable costs, and the allocation of fixed costs across the various organs. In 2005, the average organ acquisition cost per transplanted organ (kidneys, livers, pancreases, hearts, intestines, and lungs) was $33,000 and the total Medicare expenditure on organ acquisition was $500 million (USRDS 2007, 224). The standard acquisition cost also depends on the average number of organs procured per donor, which in turn depends on the proximity of transplant programs that use these organs, and the rates at which recovered organs are actually transplanted. For example, based on data reported in *Transplant Program and OPO Specific Reports* published online by the Scientific Registry of Transplant Recipients for the year ending June 30, 2007, the average number of organs recovered per donor nationally was 3.5, but ranged from 2.6 to 4.0 across OPOs; nationally, the fraction of procured kidneys actually transplanted was 0.83, but ranged from 0.65 to 0.93 across OPOs. Recovering more organs per donor reduces the share of fixed costs allocated to each organ type in the numerator of the standard acquisition charge. Increasing the percentage of organs actually transplanted increases the denominator.

Although the three primary activities of OPOs continue to be receiving referrals from hospitals, determining donor status and obtaining consent from families, and coordinating the recovery of organs by transplant surgeons, the number of organizational tasks is much larger (Mone 2002). OPOs develop protocols with hospitals and educate their staffs to ensure appropriate referrals of potential donors. They manage the medical care given to the donor once consent is received, including organizing and documenting the circumstances of recovery. They arrange placement of organs through the OPTN and submit related data. They oversee organ preservation, which may include techniques, such as pulsatile perfusion for kidneys, that may improve graft function, especially for organs from older donors (Matsuoka et al. 2006). OPOs also engage in public education both to encourage individuals to commit to donation before death and to increase the chances that families will agree to donation after death. To obtain accreditation from the Association of Organ Procurement Organizations, they must engage in a number of quality assurance activities such as periodic reviews of hospital death records to determine whether they are receiving appropriate referrals.

OPOs depend on the time and effort invested by transplant surgeons. Professional and financial interests create strong incentives for transplant surgeons to make efforts that increase the number of organs available to their own patients. Professionally, organs enable them to improve the quality and length of their patients' lives. Financially, transplants generate revenues for surgeons and their transplant centers. Indeed, they are one of the most profitable types of surgery for hospitals (Resnick et al. 2005). Because organs are the scarcest resource in the transplantation system, they are the primary source of rents to providers. In a market system, the rents would be captured by the suppliers or procurers of organs, but suppliers and procurers are legally prohibited from engaging in commercial transactions; further, OPOs are reimbursed for their costs by the federal government and required to transfer the organs they procure to transplant centers at the standard acquisition charge. The total costs of transplants are high—in 2008, the average billed charges in the United States for the thirty days before the transplant and the 180 days after for kidneys, livers, and hearts were $259,000, $523,400, and $787,700, respectively (Hauboldt and Hanson 2008, 5). As transplant centers perform more surgeries, they spread their fixed costs over more transplants so that their average costs fall. With excess demand for transplants, as evidenced by long waiting lists, the decline in average cost does not reduce the price of transplants to patients and their third-party payers, primarily the federal government. Consequently, transplant centers and their surgeons accrue rents from the organs they are allocated.

Depending on the nature of allocation, professional and personal interests may not be as closely aligned with respect to efforts to procure organs. Professionally, surgeons try to help because they realize that the organs are valuable to patients, whether their own or those of other surgeons—conservatively valuing a life-year at $100,000 leads to estimates of the net social benefits of each cadaveric donor of more than $1 million (Mendeloff et al. 2004). However, exhorting and supporting procurement efforts require commitments of time. In some cases, these commitments may be substantial, such as when a transplant surgeon must travel in the middle of the night to a remote trauma center to recover organs. The financial benefits to the surgeons depend on how the organs are allocated—specifically, the degree to which the procured organs are common property available to other transplant centers. If the organs are allocated to the procuring surgeons' patients, then these surgeons receive the full rent; if they are put into a larger pool, then the surgeons receive only a fraction of the full rent depending on the number of surgeons sharing the pool. The fewer surgeons, the more likely it is that the expected financial benefit exceeds the costs borne by the procuring surgeon. This logic becomes relevant in assessing the geographic priority of allocation as discussed in chapter 5.

A natural metric for assessing the performance of OPOs is the donation rate. The number of donors can be easily measured as can the numbers of various organs procured. So too can the numbers of organs transplanted, though these numbers reflect not only the efficiency of the OPO but also the willingness of the transplant centers to accept organs of various qualities. Measuring an appropriate base for calculating the donation rate is much more difficult. Population or total deaths are easily measured, but remain crude proxies for the potential number of donors. More appropriate data for measuring the number of potential donors can be gathered from reviews of hospital records, but at higher cost and only after some delay. Risk adjustment also poses some difficult questions. For example, should geographic extent and population density, both potentially relevant to the costs of procurement, be taken into account? Should demographic characteristics that may be relevant to the willingness of people to donate be taken into account? Should the characteristics of the hospitals in which procurement takes place be taken into account?

The problems of measurement and appropriate risk adjustment have slowed the introduction of a report card for OPOs like the one now available for transplant programs. In

January 2008, to create a better database for assessing the conversion of potential to actual donors, the OPTN began collecting data on the demographic characteristics and cause of death for each potential donor meeting eligibility requirements. Also, the SRTR has begun using these data to estimate risk-adjusted models for donation rates for selected OPOs. However, the report card that the SRTR currently makes available online (www.ustransplant.org) suppresses risk adjustment and simply reports raw donation rates, the number of deceased donors who provided at least one organ divided by the number of OPO-reported aggregate eligible deaths from hospitals. These rates vary considerably, ranging from 0.452 to 0.825, suggesting great variation in performance, the importance of risk adjustment, or both. The report card also provides data on the average number of organs per donor, the percentage of each type of recovered organ actually transplanted, and the distribution of cold ischemic times (the times between retrieval and transplant).

Efforts to Increase Donation Rates

Donated organs are the scarce resource in transplantation. Members of the transplant community, often assisted and sometimes prodded by state and federal policymakers, have made a variety of efforts to increase donation rates. As noted, states quickly adopted the Uniform Anatomical Gift Act and facilitated expressing the intention to donate when drivers' licenses are issued. Many states, at the urging of the transplantation community, followed with required request laws making OPOs responsible for approaching the families of potential donors and routine notification laws requiring hospitals to inform OPOs about potential donors; the federal government subsequently mandated routine notification (HHS 1998b). As also noted, states have taken the lead in enforcing donor intentions against the norm of deference to family wishes through first-person consent laws and the creation of donor lists.

Several states have attempted to provide financial incentives for donation. Most prominently, in 1994 Pennsylvania adopted a law that allows residents to earmark one dollar of their license registration fee for the Organ Donor Awareness Trust Fund. The law also provides for reimbursement on request for up to three thousand dollars for funeral expenses of donors whose organs are actually used, though the fund has only been large enough to allow maximum payments of three hundred dollars (Ubel et al. 2000). In 2004 Wisconsin changed its income tax law to allow living donors to deduct up to ten thousand dollars for travel and lodging expenses and lost wages associated with donation. A number of other states have since adopted similar laws. The same year, the president signed the Organ Donation and Recovery Act (Public Law 108-216), which authorized the U.S. Department of Health and Human Services (HHS) secretary to give grants to states, transplant centers, OPOs, and other organizations to reimburse live donors for travel and subsistence expenses; grants to hospitals and OPOs to fund programs coordinating organ donation activities; and grants and contracts to promote public awareness, initiate demonstration projects, and conduct evaluations.

The federal government has supported a number of initiatives by professional organizations over the years. The longest ongoing initiative is the National Minority Organ/ Tissue Transplant Education Program (MOTTEP), begun in 1993 by Howard University transplant surgeon Clive Callendar, who drew on twenty years of community outreach experience and research in the District of Columbia. MOTTEP originally focused on three cities, but received funding in 1995 from the National Institutes of Health to expand to its current coverage of fifteen cities (Callendar, Miles, and Hall 2003). Its original focus was on improving African American awareness of transplantation and the need for organ donation. It subsequently expanded its target audience to include other minorities and its mission to include disease prevention. Although there have been no systematic assessments of MOTTEP's impact on minority donation, it almost certainly has contributed to the growth in the percentage of deceased donors who are African American from 8.8 percent in 1988 to 11.2 percent in 1998 to 16 percent in 2008 (OPTN 2009). As discussed in chapter 6, these increases are especially important in light of the overrepresentation of African Americans on the kidney waiting list, and the role of genetically based factors in kidney allocation.

More recently, HHS sponsored the Organ Donation Breakthrough Collaborative to increase donation rates in large hospitals. Then Secretary Tommy Thompson, who had been a strong advocate of organ donation as governor of Wisconsin, started the Gift of Life Donation Initiative shortly after taking office. Beginning in 2003, the department worked with the nonprofit Institute for Healthcare Improvement to establish collaborative teams drawn form OPOs and their associated hospitals to achieve the goal of increasing the ratio of eligible donors to actual donors to 75 percent, a rate met in 2002 by only fifteen of the largest two hundred hospitals (Shafer et al. 2006). The collaborative looked for best practices at OPOs with high conversion rates and then worked with local teams to implement these practices, adapt them to local circumstances, and continuously assess results. By April 2004 thirty-six of the ninety-five participating hospitals participating in the first of the three collaborative efforts reached the 75 percent goal. In 2004 donations in these ninety-five hospitals increased by 16 percent over 2003, versus 9 percent in other U.S. hospitals (Shafer et al. 2006). Results from the second and third waves, which have also included some Canadian hospitals, have not yet been formally assessed.

Enlarging the Pool of Donors: Reviving Cardiac Death

The procurement of cadaveric organs requires a clear and accepted definition of death. Under common law death was defined as the cessation of all vital functions and determined by the absence of spontaneous respiratory and cardiac functions. During the 1950s ventilators that made it possible to support respiration for patients with full loss of brain function came into common use. The organs of patients receiving oxygen from ventilators remained viable and therefore potentially transplantable. Absent a clear definition of death, however, organs could not be harvested. The first initiative to create a definition that would encompass these patients was made by a committee formed at the Harvard Medical School in 1967. Its report argued for viewing the brain as the primary organ of the body and proposed as a definition the irreversible cessation of all functions of the entire brain (Harvard Medical School 1968). It thus proposed what has become known as brain death, or whole brain death, determined by total unawareness of external stimuli and unresponsiveness to painful stimuli; absence of spontaneous muscular movement, spontaneous respiration, and response to stimuli; and absence of reflex responses.

In 1980 the National Conference of Commissioners on Uniform State Laws drafted the Uniform Determination of Death Act, which was based on its own Uniform Brain Death Act and similar proposals from the American Bar Association and the American Medical Association. Section 1 of the act states that "an individual who has sustained either (1) irreversible cessation of circulatory and respiratory functions, or (2) irreversible cessation of all functions of the entire brain, including the brain stem, is dead. A determination of death must be made in accordance with accepted medical standards" (1980, 3). The Uniform Determination of Death Act was endorsed by the President's Commission for the Study of Ethical Problems in Medicine and Biomedical and Behavioral Research (1981) and has subsequently been adopted by most states and many other countries.

The introduction of the definition of brain death led to the near abandonment of procuring organs from individuals whose circulatory and respiratory functions had irreversibly ceased, what is commonly referred to as cardiac death. In 1994 only 1.1 percent of donors experienced cardiac death; by 2004 the number had risen fivefold but still was only 5.5 percent (Childress and Liverman 2006, 142). The primary reason is that organs are removed only after cardiac arrest and at least a further two to five minutes, during which the cessation of cardiopulmonary function is verified. This period adds to the warm ischemic time, the period between the cessation of circulation and the cooling of the organ in preparation for preservation. Although the warm ischemic time can potentially reduce the chances of graft success, in practice the rates of success with brain and cardiac death kidney donations appear to be comparable (Cooper et al. 2004). A national conference in 2005 sponsored by the UNOS Foundation and other organizations, and supported by analysis from SRTR staff, concluded that graft success rates were comparable for kidneys but not for livers (Bernat et al. 2006).

Donation after cardiac death also raises ethical concerns. One concern is that, with the consent of family members, life-sustaining measures are stopped before death. Another is that donation requires preparations. For example, the blood thinner heparin is often administered while the patient is still alive to reduce the chances that the capacity for blood flow into the organs will be reduced. These concerns have been addressed by three Institute of Medicine committees (Childress and Liverman 2006). The most recent committee assessed donation after cardiac death as ethically valid in controlled circumstances, that is, in settings in which the family or surrogate has decided to withdraw support measures. It noted, however, that ethical concerns still need to be addressed for the much larger pool of potential donors who experience cardiac death in uncontrolled circumstances, that is, after efforts to resuscitate have failed.

The OPTN has taken a number of steps to encourage donation after cardiac death. As discussed in chapter 6, kidneys generally go to patients on the national waiting list if they do not have genetic mismatches for key antigens. To create an incentive for recovery of kidneys after cardiac death at the local level, the rules exempt these kidneys from mandatory national sharing. Rather, they follow the local, regional, and national priority followed for kidneys that have one or more mismatches. In 2006 the Membership and Professional Standards Committee, following the recommendations made by the National

Conference on Donation after Cardiac Death, worked with the OPO Committee to develop a proposal to the board of directors that required all OPOs and transplant hospitals to develop protocols for recovering organs after cardiac death. The board approved changing the bylaws to include this requirement at its December 2006 meeting.

Enlarging the Pool of Donors: Expanded Criteria Donor Kidneys

The ideal organ donor is a healthy, young person who suffers a head injury that affects only the brain. Older donors are less than ideal in the sense that their organs have higher risks of graft failure and shorter expected longevity—even when grafts are successful, younger patients may outlive organs from older donors. (Conversely, organs from young donors transplanted into older recipients may have many years of graft function remaining when the recipient dies—a point relevant to the discussion of net benefit in chapter 7.) A number of medical conditions may also increase the risk of graft failure. Nonetheless, the pressing shortage of organs has led OPOs increasingly to seek organs from older and less healthy patients, referred to as expanded criteria donors (ECDs). An offer of one of these ECD organs poses a difficult dilemma for patients and their transplant surgeons: either accept a less than ideal organ or wait an indefinite time for a better organ. Many of the organs from older and less healthy donors were being rejected and ultimately discarded. In 2001, for instance, the proportion of ultimately discarded standard criteria kidneys was about 8 percent, compared to about 40 percent for kidneys meeting what has become the operational definition of ECD (Metzger et al. 2003, 116).

In 2001 the American Society of Transplantation and the American Society of Transplant Surgeons sponsored a meeting to develop guidelines for improving the recovery and transplantation of cadaveric organs (Rosengard et al. 2002). Seeking to reduce the discarding of recovered organs from older donors, the Kidney Work Group proposed that kidneys from all donors over age sixty be allocated solely on the basis of waiting time among patients who, after being informed of the additional risks, voluntarily agreed to be placed on a list of patients consenting to accept these kidneys. The OPTN Organ Availability Committee and the Kidney and Pancreas Committee, which had been seeking to define ECD kidneys, took up the proposal. The committees decided to seek an operational definition of ECD kidneys such that these kidneys would have a relative risk of graft failure greater than 1.7 compared to healthy donors between the ages of ten and thirty-nine. Based on analyses done by the SRTR staff, the committees identified combinations of four risk factors—age, cerebrovascular accident (stroke) as cause of death, history of hypertension, and predonation creatinine level above 1.5 milligrams per deciliter—that produced relative risks greater than the 1.7 threshold. Specifically, they defined ECD kidneys as coming from two age groups: donors sixty or older and donors between fifty and fifty-nine who had two or more of the three risk factors. The OPTN board of directors adopted this definition in November 2001.

The board also adopted an allocation policy along the lines proposed by the Kidney Working Group. A list of suitable candidates was established. If a candidate and an ECD kidney have zero mismatches for the relevant genetic antigens, then the transplant center listing that patient is given two hours to decide whether or not to accept it. If the center does not accept the kidney, then it is released to the OPO that procured it for allocation to a local patient based on time on the suitable candidate list. If the kidney is not accepted for a local patient, then it is offered first regionally and then nationally according to time on the suitable candidate list.

The ECD kidney allocation policy went into effect on October 31, 2002. In June 2004, to encourage further the acceptance of ECD kidneys, the board of directors removed these organs from the payback requirement for accepted zero mismatched kidneys: centers that accepted zero mismatched kidneys for their patients incur an obligation to eventually pay back the OPOs that procured them with their locally procured kidneys. An analysis comparing the use of ECD kidneys in the eighteen months just before implementation of the initial allocation policy with the first eighteen months following it showed mixed results (Sung et al. 2005). Although the discard rate remained unchanged, the percentage of both recovered and transplanted ECD cadaveric kidneys went up. Subsequent analysis found wide variation across transplant centers in terms of the percentage of patients placed on the ECD list and a substantial increase in the proportion of those older than sixty-five receiving ECD transplants (Schold et al. 2006). A study at one major transplant center found that, because ECD kidneys involve a higher risk of delayed graft function requiring longer hospital stays, their greater use may reduce the profitability of kidney programs, perhaps hindering efforts for further expansion (Englesbe et al. 2008). The authors suggest that Medicare reimbursement should be risk adjusted to remove any disincentive to use ECD kidneys.

The dichotomous distinction between standard and ECD kidneys has a number of limitations (Freeman and Klintmalm 2006). These include the arbitrary choice of a 1.7 relative risk ratio, a limited set of risk factors in classification, obscured overlap in the distributions of relative risks, and contribution to the view among the public of ECD kidneys as inferior organs. As discussed in chapter 7, the proposal to revise the entire kidney allocation system would replace the dichotomous classification of standard and ECD kidneys with a continuous scale integrated into a unified allocation system.

Live Donation

With about thirty-four thousand people being added to the kidney waiting list annually, in the absence of live donations, more than seventeen thousand cadaveric donors, each providing two kidneys, would be needed each year just to keep the waiting list from growing. The number of cadaveric donors required would be lower, about fourteen thousand, if current numbers of live donations continued. Nonetheless, the number of cadaveric donations would still have to more than double to keep pace with the growing demand for kidney transplants as baby boomers age and the greater morbidity risks associated with higher prevalence of obesity increase the number of people with end-stage renal disease (ESRD). Consequently, with the technology currently available, only large increases in the rates of live donation would substantially reduce the length of the kidney transplant waiting list.

Live donation has always been common for kidneys: the natural endowment of two kidneys allows one to be donated at minimal risk to the donor. In 1988, when comprehensive statistics first became available through the SRTR, 31.9 percent of kidney donors were alive. The proportion of live donors peaked at 52.9 percent in 2003. In 2007 the rate was 45.5 percent, with just over six thousand live donors (OPTN 2009).

Live donations of liver and lung lobes are also possible, though they involve somewhat greater risk and inconvenience to the donor. The percentage of liver transplants from live donors did not reach 1 percent until 1992 and in 2007 had risen to only 3.7 percent (266 donors). The percentage of lung transplants from live donors reached 1 percent in 1991, rose to a high of 6.9 percent in 1999, and fell to 0.4 percent (only six donors) by 2007. These declines partly reflect much greater success in recovering cadaveric donations: between 2000 and 2007 the number of transplanted cadaveric livers rose from approximately five thousand to seven thousand and the number of transplanted cadaveric lungs from 825 to almost fourteen hundred (OPTN 2009). Much of the declines in recent years in the percentages of donations from live donors are thus due to increases in cadaveric donation, resulting at least in part from the success of the Organ Donation Breakthrough Collaborative.

The National Organ Transplantation Act did not explicitly give the OPTN a role in overseeing live donation. Although live kidney donation was common at the time, it generally involved transplant centers facilitating donations from relatives, spouses, or close friends, transactions in turn involving augmentation of total supply rather than allocation of the very limited supply of cadaveric organs. Transplant centers made their own choices about how aggressively to promote live donation and developed their own policies to ensure that live donations were truly voluntary and based on informed consent. For example, transplant centers keep the medical acceptability of donor candidates confidential and report incompatibility for candidates who do not wish to be donors for any reason.

Transplantation of live-donor rather than deceased-donor kidneys is usually medically preferable for patients for three reasons. First, the graft success rate is generally higher. For transplants done during 2002 through 2004, the one-year graft survival rate in the United States was 89 percent for deceased-donor kidneys and 95.1 percent for live-donor kidneys. For transplants from 1999 through 2002, the three-year survival rates were 77.8 for deceased-donor and 87.8 for live-donor kidneys; for 1997 through 2000, the five-year rates were 66.5 percent for deceased-donor and 79.7 percent for live-donor kidneys (OPTN 2009). Second, live donation often allows transplants to be done earlier than they would be if patients wait for cadaveric kidneys. This is especially valuable for children, who suffer developmentally from dialysis, and for patients, like most diabetics, who do not tolerate dialysis well. Preemptive transplants, those before the initiation of dialysis, are especially valuable in preserving health status for these patients. Third, the opportunity to plan transplants from live donors may reduce the stress patients suffer from the uncertainty about if and when a cadaveric kidney will become available.

Simply having a loved one or friend willing to donate a kidney does not guarantee that the patient will receive a live-donor transplant. As explained in chapter 6, a number of factors such as blood type and sensitization to various antigens may preclude a patient from receiving a kidney from any particular donor, live or deceased. In these situations, which occur in almost one-third of cases, a patient may have to forgo live-donor kidney transplantation from the willing donor. Of course, if and when these patients receive deceased-donor kidneys, they deny the kidneys they receive to others on the waiting list who would have received them had the live-donor kidney transplants gone forward.

One way around the problem of willing but incompatible living donors is to facilitate paired donation, an idea proposed more than two decades ago (Rapaport 1986). Paired donation links a pair of incompatible donor-patient dyads such that both donors are compatible with the patients in the other dyads to which they were paired. Liane Friedman Ross and colleagues proposed an ethical framework for a paired-kidney-exchange program (1997). About this time, transplant professionals in the Washington, DC metropolitan area and UNOS Region 1 (New England) began working to develop plans for implementing paired exchanges. They expanded the idea to include list-exchange donations, in which an incompatible live donor provides a kidney to the kidney transplant waiting list in return for that donor's intended recipient receiving higher priority for a cadaveric kidney. Because list exchanges involve cadaveric organs, it was necessary for the Washington Regional Transplant Community, the OPO for the Washington, DC area, and Region 1 to obtain variances from the OPTN. Thus, for the first time, the OPTN became directly involved in policies related to live donation.

In 1999 the OPTN board of directors approved the variance for the Washington Regional Voluntary Living Donor Registry, which was implemented in January 2000, and in 2000 the variance for the Region 1 list-exchange and paired-donor program, which was implemented in February 2001. The variances require transplant centers first to seek to match pairs of incompatible donor-patient dyads for exchanges before turning to list exchanges. The list exchanges involve the donated kidney being allocated to the waiting list as if it were a deceased-donor kidney and then the original intended recipient of the live donation receiving rights of first refusal for cadaveric kidneys as they become available within the local area until a transplant is made. By the end of 2003, four paired exchanges and seventeen list exchanges had been made in Region 1 (Delmonico et al. 2004). The Washington Regional Voluntary Living Donor Registry produced ten paired exchanges and ten list exchanges by March 2004 (Gilbert et al. 2005).

List exchanges have not been widely embraced for a number of practical and ethical concerns (Ross and Zenios 2004). Most important, because the live donors are usually blood types A and B, they cannot donate to type O patients. (If the live donors were type O, they could—absent sensitivity—have donated to any blood type, including their intended recipients.) Consequently, type O patients may have to wait longer than they would have had the list exchange not been made.

In contrast, paired exchange programs have been widely embraced. The capacity for these programs to make the appropriate matches depends on the number of donor-patient dyads among which to search for compatible pairs. It also depends on the development of algorithms that allow for the rapid identification of possible pairs and the expansion of matching opportunities to higher order exchanges involving more than a single pair (Saidman et al. 2006). Some regional networks, such as the New England Program for Kidney Exchange, have formed to expand the pools of possible exchanges. Creating a national pool involving all transplant centers offers the greatest potential for more and better matches (Segev et al. 2005).

In July 2004 the OPTN Kidney Transplantation Committee developed a concept for a national paired exchange program for kidneys. The committee identified the need to specify data requirements for listing incompatible donor-patient dyads, to address the logistical issues involved in carrying out the paired exchanges, including a matching algorithm, and to determine the required donor and patient follow-up requirements. It issued the concept for public comment and discussion by the regions. Because the comments and regional feedback were overwhelmingly positive, the board of directors voted to endorse the concept at its November 2004 meeting. Concerns about whether paired exchanges involved a transfer of organs with a valuable consideration, and hence were illegal under the National Organ Transplant Act, however, prompted the board to defer implementation until the concerns could be allayed. At its November 2005 meeting, the board adopted a motion to ask HHS to assist it in efforts to obtain a legislative resolution of the concerns. In the meantime, the Kidney Transplant Committee formed a working group, which included many people with experience in various local and regional paired exchange programs already under way, to help develop a more specific concept proposal that could be sent out for comment when legal concerns were resolved.

Resolution of the concerns about illegality came from two sources. First, the Office of Legal Counsel at the Department of Justice issued a memorandum that neither paired nor list exchanges were illegal under the National Organ Transplant Act (Marshall 2007). Second, Congress passed legislation (Public Law 110-144) at the end of 2007 that amended the National Organ Transplant Act to make paired exchanges explicitly legal.

Although the OPTN is developing a national program, many of the local and regional programs are extending their efforts beyond simple paired exchanges to those involving three or four donor-patient dyads. Some programs have also begun to implement chain, or domino, donations. The chain begins with an altruistic, or undirected, live donation. The undirected donation goes to a patient in an incompatible donor-patient dyad and the donor in that dyad makes a donation to another incompatible dyad, and so forth, until the donor in the last appropriate dyad makes an undirected donation to the kidney waiting list. The longest such chain implemented by the end of 2008 was executed by surgeons at Johns Hopkins Hospital and involved six kidneys (Dominguez 2008). Of course, one could imagine seeding chains with a cadaveric kidney and repaying the list with a kidney from the last living donor in the chain. Like list exchanges, however, such chains raise difficult issues because the person on the list who forgoes the initial cadaveric kidney will not necessarily be an appropriate recipient for the live donation returned at the end of the chain. Consequently, chains beginning with a cadaveric kidney would require an explicit OPTN variance.

At the direction of the HHS Office of Transplantation, the OPTN has begun to develop guidelines and data requirements related to live donation (Burdick 2004). For example, transplant centers currently report any deaths of living donors, their return to the operating room in the postoperative period, their rehospitalization within six months of the donation, and any organ failures they suffer that require them to be put on the transplant waiting list (Delmonico and Graham 2006). Subsequently, at the request of the OPTN, HHS undertook a rulemaking to clarify that OPTN policies related to living donation would have the same legal status as its policies concerning the procurement and allocation of cadaveric organs (HHS 2006a). That is, data reporting requirements would be legally binding but other policies would be enforced through membership standing.

Reconsidering Markets?

Medical ethicists have helped build what Mark Cherry calls a "global consensus" that organ markets should be prohibited because they create financial incentives that coerce the poor, violate human dignity, promote greater inequality between rich and poor, undercut the desirable exercise of altruism, and, following Titmuss, result in poorer quality organs being transplanted and therefore worse medical outcomes (2005, 4–5). Nonetheless, a number of other ethicists have made arguments in favor of markets on a variety of grounds, ranging from respect for personal autonomy to utilitarianism (Dworkin 1994; Taylor 2005). The more recent of these writers argued that the morality of organ markets cannot be assessed in the abstract, but must rather be determined in terms of the specifics of their regulation. In other words, they urged an assessment of all the morally relevant consequences of concrete alternatives, something widely recognized as an important practice of good policy analysis (Weimer and Vining 2005).

Although markets for cadaveric donations elicit less convincing moral objections than markets for live donors do, they face a number of practical problems that limit their attractiveness. Although some argue for spot markets in which private agents would attempt to purchase rights to organs from the families of the recently deceased (Kaserman and Barnett 2002), the more plausible proposals involve futures markets, in which a living person promises a donation upon death in return for a payment at the time of promise. The name of the future donor would be added to a national list that would be consulted by hospitals when patients face imminent death. A futures market along these general lines was first suggested by Richard Schwindt and Aidan Vining (1986). The payment would be made by either a private entity, such as by a health insurer at a market-determined price, or by a government agency at an administered price. In the case of the private entity as purchaser, the compensation it would receive when organs are actually recovered would almost certainly have to be set administratively. In either case, the supply and demand side of the markets would effectively be separated so that individual patients would not be purchasing organs but rather receiving purchased organs through the existing allocation systems. Whereas an administered spot price could be reasonably set based on either the net social benefits or the net fiscal savings of a typical kidney transplant relative to dialysis, the determination of an appropriate futures price would be quite complicated, in that it would require actuarial assessments of the likelihood of a death that would produce a useable organ and the timing of that death.

A market for live-donor kidneys would almost certainly have to be a spot market, and therefore would avoid the problem of relating futures prices to current prices. As with the market for cadaveric donors, to be politically viable the supply and demand sides of the live-donor market would surely have to be separated for it to avoid objections that it would promote the exploitation of the poor by the rich. Currently, steps are taken to ensure that altruistic donors are fully informed, acting voluntarily, and appropriately motivated psychologically. Comparable steps would be required to vet those who sell their kidneys, though the bounds of appropriate motivation would be more difficult to determine. For example, would immediate fiscal distress be an appropriate motivation?

Short of the creation of a sanctioned market for organs, the OPTN will most likely confront issues related to private efforts to obtain live donations. For example, recently a nonprofit organization incorporated in New York state, the National Kidney Registry, began providing assistance to incompatible donor-patient dyads seeking exchanges as well as information to patients about how to recruit living donors. To what extent should transplant centers participate in the recruitment of live donors for paired exchanges or altruistic donations? A recent study estimated that about 5 percent of transplants worldwide are done commercially in a country other than that of the patient (Shimazono 2007, 959). The OPTN board of directors went on record in opposition to such transplant tourism in 2006. What responsibilities should transplant centers have for patients who do travel overseas to purchase transplants either legally or in black markets? Should these patients have access to cadaveric organs if their grafts fail?

Conclusion

Organs remain the scarce resource in transplantation. Increasing the availability of transplant organs offers large benefits for patients and society—they permit longer and healthier lives. Increasing the supply of kidneys even reduces total federal expenditures on the treatment of ESRD. Not only those involved in transplantation as professionals, patients, and their families, but also much of the general public and many politicians, recognize that these benefits cannot be realized without donated organs. It is not surprising that the OPTN has played both a general role in the widespread efforts to increase organ supply as well as a specific role through the modification of allocation rules relevant to the donation and effective use of transplant organs.

Organ donation raises important ethical concerns related to autonomy, consent, and human dignity, especially for donations from the living. Altruism continues to be the organizing principle for the U.S. organ supply system. Although it need not conflict with autonomy, its promotion through the creation of opportunity for the families of the deceased to act altruistically may very well have reduced the number of recovered organs, and therefore lives saved. States that have adopted first-person consent laws appear to believe that this is the case. One can also wonder if the growing transplant waiting lists will eventually result in a balancing of altruism with utilitarianism through greater use of incentives and perhaps even highly regulated markets.

OPTN policies that promote greater availability of transplant organs are positive sum in the sense that all involved in transplantation benefit. In contrast, OPTN policies that determine the allocation of the limited supply of cadaveric organs are effectively zero sum in the sense that if one person receives a transplant organ then another cannot. The next three chapters consider how the OPTN makes decisions regarding these more challenging zero-sum policies.

5

Liver Allocation and the Final Rule

The National Organ Transplant Act of 1984 transformed the voluntary network of organizations involved in solid organ transplantation into a formal network with effectively mandatory membership and governance by the OPTN. Since it began operations in 1986, the OPTN has exercised de facto authority over the content of rules governing the procurement and allocation of cadaveric organs. The de jure basis of this authority was disputed throughout the 1990s, but especially between 1994 and 2000, when HHS, which has oversight responsibility for the OPTN, developed and finalized rules that sought to impose specific allocation criteria on the OPTN and subject it to stronger oversight. The extended controversy over this rulemaking, which was inextricably intertwined with liver allocation policies, provides a window for viewing both the role of the OPTN in federal governance as well as OPTN internal decision making. In other words, it provides an excellent opportunity for observing how private rulemaking functions as a medical governance arrangement in its political context.

Several aspects of cadaveric liver allocation make it particularly useful as a perspective on private regulation. First, cadaveric livers are extremely valuable goods. In contrast to kidney failure, which can be treated by either dialysis or transplantation, fulminant liver failure means imminent death if a transplant is not possible. Further, in contrast to kidneys, whose double endowment makes live donations readily feasible and fairly common, livers for transplants are overwhelmingly cadaveric—transplants involving partial livers from live donors in 2008 accounted for only 3.6 percent of donations (OPTN 2009). Because cadaveric donations remain the primary source for transplant livers, their allocation is very consequential for patients, often a matter of life and death.

Second, liver allocation has direct implications for the ability of transplant centers to serve their patients, and hence to promote their own professional and financial interests. Between 1990 and 2001 the number of centers performing liver transplants increased from 74 to 116, and the number doing more than 10 transplants per year increased from 52 to 98 (UNOS 2003, table 9.10). As more centers began doing liver transplants, a larger fraction of cadaveric organs stayed in the local areas where they were procured. In 2001, 63 percent of liver transplants involved organs procured locally, up from 39 percent in 1990 (UNOS 2000, table 25; 2003, table 37). With average billed charges of hundreds of thousands of dollars per liver transplant, the financial consequences for transplant centers and surgeons of even small shifts in transplant volumes are substantial.

Third, liver transplantation has been advancing rapidly, providing a stimulus to reconsider the scientific basis of rules already in place. Particularly relevant to geographic sharing is cold ischemic time, the time organs are viable after being procured. The growing use of partial organs and the splitting of cadaveric organs among multiple recipients will in time likely lead to revised rules. Such changes, and the difficulty in assessing them scientifically, imply that considerable expertise is needed to predict and evaluate the consequences of allocation rules. Thus the normative assessment of liver allocation rules involves expertise as well as values.

Fourth, controversy over the appropriate role of geography in liver allocation expanded to include debate over the role that HHS oversight should play in shaping organ allocation rules more generally. HHS efforts to move the OPTN toward less geographically based liver allocation shows both the potential influence and inherent limitations of its oversight role.

This chapter does not attempt to resolve the normative issue of the extent to which geography should be a factor in liver allocation for two reasons. First, uncertainty remains around the answers to many relevant questions about impacts: To what extent would wider geographic sharing result in more lives, life-years, or quality-adjusted life-years saved? Would better matching of patients to livers result? Would longer cold ischemic times result in less graft success? Would graft success increase if more livers went to higher volume centers? Would fewer livers be procured if transplant centers kept fewer livers for their own use? What groups of patients, if any, would be disadvantaged?

Second, the values that should be applied in assessing these effects are not clear. The legal framework calls for the application of medical criteria. Should these criteria be specified in an attempt to maximize the number of lives immediately saved by allocating livers to those who face imminent death, or the gains in life-years or quality-adjusted life-years by allocating livers to those who would obtain the largest marginal gains? Should the distributional consequences, to patients or to transplant centers, be considered in choosing medical criteria? Disagreement over and uncertainty about these questions, along with stakeholder interests, sets the stage for controversy.

Rather, this chapter considers the operation of private rulemaking and its oversight. In broad outline, the controversy involved HHS's attempting to eliminate local priority in the allocation rules established by UNOS, the OPTN contractor, for transplant organs generally, but most immediately for livers. The controversy involved vocal critics of the existing allocation system seeking to secure a major change in its operation, an extended rulemaking by HHS, congressional intercession, and efforts by a number of states to maintain local priority in allocation. Ultimately, HHS relaxed the specificity of its proposed rule and the OPTN made revisions in liver allocation that moved the system toward regional over local priority in sharing. The immense regulatory docket and other documentary sources that amassed during the controversy provide a unique window on the politics of allocation.

Controversy over Liver Allocation Rules

More than any other issue, the role of geography in allocation has been central in debates over the appropriate goals of organ allocation rules. Why so? Recall that UNOS, hence the OPTN, evolved from a voluntary association of procurement organizations and transplant centers that wished to secure gains for patients from sharing procured organs that could not be well used locally. Indeed, it was only with the creation of the OPTN that the regime moved from sharing to allocation. Further, relatively short cold ischemic times for livers and hearts, and the detailed testing needed to match kidneys, argued for a priority to local use in the initially developed allocation rules. So too did the belief that local transplant communities would make greater efforts to procure organs when their patients had priority for those organs—a belief, as discussed in chapter 4, consistent with the common property problem that arises when transplant centers do not keep all the organs that they procure. The opening of more transplant centers made it possible for more patients to receive transplants near where they live, but also diverted organs from established programs to the new ones. This diversion was especially significant for liver transplants.

Overview of Liver Allocation Rules through mid-1996

Before 1986, the informal sharing procedures employed by UNOS members were supplemented with UNOS/STAT, a rule through which a transplant center could request that notices be sent to the then approximately sixty organ procurement organizations (OPOs) indicating that a patient required a liver within twenty-four hours to survive. The first general system, adopted by UNOS for the OPTN in 1986 (Edwards and Harper 1996), was designed by Thomas Starzl of the University of Pittsburgh Medical Center (UPMC), the leading liver transplant facility (Burdick 1996). It established six levels of medical urgency in addition to the UNOS/STAT designation. Livers were allocated to patients in descending order of their medical urgency, first within the local area where they were procured, second within the region, and third nationwide. Local could be as small an area as one served by a single transplant center or as large as one served by a group of centers working together. At the time local OPOs were organized into nine regions. Within each medical urgency category, a point system based on blood type compatibility, waiting time, and logistical factors (distance between transplant center and donor location and distance between potential recipient and transplant center) determined priority.

In 1991 the UNOS/STAT designation was eliminated and the most urgent category was expanded. Many OPTN members involved in liver transplantation believed that, in the absence of formal rules governing its use, UNOS/STAT was being abused. As many as 15 percent of patients receiving liver transplants between 1987 and 1990 obtained organs under this designation (Edwards and Harper 1996, 3). It also appeared that several transplant centers were routinely using the designation for patients with less urgent chronic, rather than more urgent acute, liver failure. After an extended policy debate involving the Liver Subcommittee of the Organ Procurement and Distribution Committee and the full committee, the OPTN board of directors, which was identical to the UNOS board of directors, dropped the UNOS/STAT designation in favor of expanding the most urgent category to include patients, whether suffering from acute or chronic liver disease, who were expected to die within seven days without a transplant. At the time, only two transplant centers objected to the change (Edwards and Harper 1996, 4).

The OPTN made a number of additional modifications to the allocation system over the next four years. With respect to its basic geography, the OPTN defined the local area so that it would be no smaller than the area served by an OPO, expanded the number of regions from nine to eleven, and dropped the points awarded for closeness of potential transplant recipients and to donated organs. The number of categories of medical urgency was reduced from six to four, and points for waiting time for patients in the highest category of medical emergency were changed to be based on time in category rather than time on list. Table 5–1 summarizes the liver allocation system as it had evolved through mid-1996

Table 5–1   Liver Allocation Rules, June 1996

Patient status
1. Patient in hospital intensive care unit due to acute or chronic liver failure with life expectancy without a liver transplant of seven days: patients in status 1 automatically revert to status 2 after seven days; may be returned to status 1 by attending physician
2. Patient continuously hospitalized in an acute care bed for at least five days, or is bound for intensive care unit
3. Patient requires continuous medical care, but is not continuously hospitalized
4. Patient at home and functioning normally; transplant considered elective surgery

Geographic-status priority
1. Local patients (transplant centers in OPO where organ procured)
   A. Status 1 patients in descending order of points
   B. Status 2 patients in descending order of points
   C. Status 3 or 4 in descending order of points
2. Regional patients (transplant centers in region of OPO where organ procured)
   A. Status 1 patients in descending order of points
   B. Status 2 patients in descending order of points
   C. Status 3 or 4 in descending order of points
3. National patients
   A. Status 1 patients in descending order of points
   B. Status 2 patients in descending order of points
   C. Status 3 or 4 in descending order of points

Priority points
Up to 10 points for waiting time
Up to 10 points blood type compatibility
Points by status: status 3, 12 points; status 4, 6 points

Source: Adapted from Edwards and Harper 1996.

Stakeholder Conflict in the Regulatory Arena

The 1994 HHS notice of proposed rulemaking received a cool reception from OPTN members, with the vast majority of transplant centers favoring maintaining the governance of the OPTN with minimal federal oversight. The situation changed dramatically in 1996, however, when the OPTN board of directors voted to adopt a major revision of the liver allocation system that would lower the priority of status 1 patients with chronic liver failure. The political effect of the OPTN decision was to enable transplant centers disadvantaged by the geographically based allocation rule to mobilize opposition from chronic liver failure patients to the downgrading of status and to open a public forum for more general discussion of liver allocation.

The original motivations for the geographical basis of liver allocation included relatively short acceptable cold ischemic times for livers (about twelve hours, compared to about twenty-four hours for kidneys) and a desire by transplant surgeons to inspect livers before transplantation. As preservation technology improved, cold ischemic time became less of a constraint. In the late 1980s the geographic structure of the liver-transplant sector began changing dramatically. Many liver transplant surgeons trained at UPMC started liver transplant programs in areas of the country that previously had not had them. As a consequence, livers that in the past were exported from these areas began to be kept for local use. The number of liver transplant operations performed at the UPMC declined from 471 in 1990 to 177 in 1996, for example. As more organs were kept locally, substantial differences in waiting times across OPOs and regions appeared. For instance, one study based on data from 1990 to 1992 found that the median waiting times for patients varied across regions from a low of thirty-one days to a high of 207 (Klassen et al. 1998, 285).

Opponents of the geographically based system, including surgeons at the UPMC, argued against it on fairness grounds. Patients' priorities should depend on medical criteria only, not on which centers have listed them—patients in lower medical status categories would sometimes receive livers instead of patients in higher medical status categories in other OPOs. Patients living near each other but on opposite sides of an OPO boundary could have radically different chances of receiving an organ even though they had comparable medical conditions: relatively healthy candidates might receive livers while much sicker patients in another locale continued waiting. The disparities induced some patients to list with more than one transplant center. Some opponents noted studies indicating higher mortality rates at transplant centers with low volumes of procedures, suggesting that more lives would be saved if transplants were done at higher-volume centers (see UNOS 1994a; Edwards et al. 1999), though this criticism was muted because of the political expediency of countering the argument that national sharing would result in the closure of low-volume centers.

Proponents of the geographically based system countered with a number of arguments. National sharing would threaten the survival of smaller transplant centers that provide access for patients who would otherwise have to bear substantial costs to travel to larger centers. Local priority increases transplant survival rates by reducing the time from donation to transplant, and reduces overall transplant system costs by reducing the costs of transporting organs. Further, priority for local allocation contributes to higher rates of procurement by encouraging the local transplant community to make extra efforts to obtain organs that will go first to any appropriate local patients.

The relevant committees of the OPTN were aware of these arguments and looked for ways to make incremental changes in the existing allocation system to reduce geographic disparities. In 1993 the UMPC contracted with the CONSAD Research Corporation to develop a simulation model that would allow assessment of alternative liver allocation rules, including fully national allocation. In 1995 UNOS, prompted by discussions with HHS, contracted with the Pritsker Corporation to develop its own simulation model. The Liver and Intestinal Transplantation Committee considered results from the models for a number of representative scenarios including the UPMC proposal. In June 1996 the Liver and Intestinal Transplantation Committee and the Allocation Advisory Committee recommended to the board of directors a number of changes in the liver allocation rules, most important of which were redefining Status 1 to include only patients with acute liver failure, moving chronic patients who previously were in status 1 to status 2, and eliminating status 4; and introducing regional as opposed to local allocation for status 1 patients, where the region would be defined as the 20 percent of status 1 and status 2 patients on the regional list closest to the location where the organ was procured.

The removal of chronic patients from status 1 was motivated in part by a desire to give priority to those suffering acute episodes such as adverse reactions to therapeutic drugs. The Liver and Intestinal Transplantation Committee believed that the change would result in a net saving of lives, largely because acute patients were less likely than chronic patients to require re-transplants. Additionally, many saw making the status categories more clearly defined and more homogeneous as an essential prerequisite for moving away from local priority in allocation. Separating acute from chronic patients was seen as a first step in this process.

In November 1996, after obtaining comments on the proposed changes through public hearings, the board of directors voted to accept the revisions of the status categories. However, it rejected the proposal for regional sharing. The status revisions were to become effective as of January 1997.

Response to 1996 Call for Comments

On November 13, 1996, HHS reopened the docket for comments related to its 1994 proposed rulemaking noting that the liver allocation rule changes approved by the OPTN board of directors had "generated considerable controversy within the transplant community" (1996, 58159). The department requested comments specifically on liver allocation and organ donation. In addition to soliciting written comments, it invited participation in a public hearing to be held the following month.

The hearing appears to have been initiated in response to a request from President Bill Clinton to HHS Secretary Donna Shalala that the department review organ allocation policies (Daubert 1998, 461). Clinton's intervention, in turn, seems to have been prompted by an impassioned plea from a longtime friend and campaign contributor who happened to have financial ties to the UPMC (Weiss 1996).

The three-day hearing was held from December 10 to December 12, 1996. More than one hundred witnesses testified, and, excluding petitions and form letters, more than six hundred letters were submitted to the docket. Table 5–2 summarizes the opinions expressed. The first row reports the positions expressed in testimony by, and letters from, physicians, most of whom were associated with transplant centers or professional organizations. A large majority (89.5 percent) favored the new OPTN policy and an even larger majority (98.6 percent) opposed the government making allocation policy. The second row shows similar, if less extreme, patterns of opinion expressed by other health professionals. The third row, which reports opinions by patients and their families, shows a very different pattern. Most striking, a majority (68.8 percent) of opinions opposed the new OPTN policy on grounds that it was unfair to those with chronic disease. As shown in the fourth row, a majority of petition signatures (largely from patients and their families solicited by transplant centers) also opposed the new OPTN policy, but more because it kept local allocation than because of the status change of chronic patients. Interestingly, despite the majority of opinions expressed against the new OPTN policy, opinions expressed in testimony and letters from patients and their families and in petitions overwhelmingly opposed the federal government making allocation policy. Among the thirty national organizations that testified (not separately shown in table 5–2), nine testified in favor of the new OPTN policy and ten against it; two testified in favor of a stronger government role and ten against it.

One consequence of the hearings was that the OPTN board of directors put the changes to the liver allocation on hold and permitted two regions to experiment with broader sharing of livers for acute patients. In June 1997, however, the board adopted a status classification similar to that adopted the previous November. Status 1 was limited to acute patients with life expectancies without transplant of fewer than seven days; status 2A

Table 5–2   Responses to HHS 1996

Responses	New OPTN Policy			Stronger Government Role	
	Favor	Oppose (chronic disease)	Oppose (local allocation)	Favor	Oppose
Physicians, letters, and testimony	136 (89.5)	5 (3.3)	11 (7.2)	4 (1.4)	281 (98.6)
Other health professionals, letters, and testimony	13 (72.2)	3 (16.7)	2 (11.1)	1 (3.3)	29 (96.7)
Patients and families, letters, and testimony	31 (16.7)	128 (68.8)	27 (14.5)	2 (9.5)	19 (90.5)
Petition signatures	1,582 (20.1)	2,815 (35.7)	3,485 (44.2)	14 (1.6)	843 (98.4)

Source: Adapted from Frankel 1997.
Note: Percentages of total responses in parentheses.

comprised chronic liver failure patients in intensive care units with life expectancies of fewer than seven days, and any one of several specific conditions; status 2B comprised patients requiring continuous medical care, and any one of several specific conditions; and status 3 comprised patients requiring continuous medical care. As with the earlier allocation system, livers would be allocated by status, first locally, then regionally, and last nationally.

Another consequence of the hearing was that it encouraged HHS to require the OPTN to develop less geographically based allocation rules. Both UNOS and the UPMC invested substantially in campaigns in support of their positions. The UPMC alone spent $260,000 to lobby Congress in the two years before July 1998 (Moore 1998, 1631).

Response to the Final Rule

In April 1998, HHS published its Final Rule with a call for further comment. The rule dealt generally with its oversight of the OPTN, and specifically called for the OPTN to revise its liver allocation rule (1998a). Section 121.8(a)(3)(i) was intended to apply to all organ allocation: "Neither place of residence nor place of listing shall be a major determinant of access to a transplant." The rule called for the OPTN to give priority to creating a new liver allocation system:

> The OPTN is required to develop proposals for new allocation policies (except for livers) within a year of the effective date of the final rule. In the case of liver allocation policies, where policy development work has been underway for several years, the OPTN is required to develop a new proposed allocation policy within 60 days of the effective date. (16297)

The sixty-day requirement is very short in light of the complexity of the task; it would be totally unrealistic for any federal regulatory agency to undertake such a task so quickly. Complicating things further, the Final Rule also included a grandfather clause: the new allocation system to be devised by the OPTN was required to include a transition plan that, to the greatest extent feasible, treated those already on the national waiting list no less favorably then they would be treated under current rules.

The Final Rule gave a fairly long justification for national sharing. It presented simulation results from both the Pritsker and CONSAD simulation models (HHS 1998a, 16324–327). The Pritsker model showed a larger sum of pre- and posttransplant deaths under national sharing than under either the 1996 policy or the one proposed by the Allocation Committee; it also showed national sharing offering a higher total of life years for patients than the 1996 policy but less than the policy proposed by the Allocation Committee. The CONSAD model, in contrast, showed national sharing dominating the other two allocation rules in terms of both total deaths and life years. HHS noted the differences in assumptions in these models and various factors that neither model included, such as changes in graft survival rates resulting from transplants to different types of patients and organ wastage resulting from transportation. Because the models showed only small differences in deaths and life years of national versus local sharing, the department argued that the greater equity of national sharing could be obtained without significant losses in terms of these measures of the aggregate performance of the allocation system.

The debate on the impacts of national sharing continued in the medical journals. For example, the case for national sharing and the Final Rule was presented in the *New England Journal of Medicine* (Ubel and Caplan 1998). Opponents argued that more deaths would result because of longer storage times in transit, which would reduce graft and patient survival rates and necessitate more re-transplants, and that the sickest first principle as applied in national allocation would, in the presence of the great shortage of organs, force many patients to suffer long periods of decline and morbidity risk before they gained access to transplants (Turcotte 1999). Others pointed to the harm the expected closure of smaller transplant centers would cause to medically disadvantaged patients who would be financially unable to seek transplants at other centers (Rabkin 1999).

An examination of the docket reveals that letters were sent by physicians associated with eighty-five transplant centers. Table 5–3 presents the distribution of these letters in terms of the opinion expressed on the liver rule (national allocation) and the proposed increased role for HHS in overseeing the development of OPTN policies. As with the 1996 testimony and letters, a large majority of transplant centers (forty-eight against, seven for) opposed the greater role. An even larger majority (fifty-eight against, seven for) opposed the proposal for national allocation of livers. Confirming the clear visual impression, the common tests for independence (Fisher's exact test, Tau-b, gamma) strongly reject the hypothesis that there is no relationship between the two opinions.

Table 5–4 compares several characteristics of transplant centers conditional on the opinions expressed in their letters. (For comparison, the middle row of the table shows the characteristics for centers that did not submit letters to the docket—they are on average smaller in terms of total number of transplants than those centers that submitted letters. In a logistic regression predicting probability of submitting a letter, total volume of transplants is a statistically significant predictor.) The first three rows consider opinions related to the HHS role. The group opposing a greater role had roughly the same market share of liver transplants in 1998 as in 1990, whereas those either not expressing an opinion or expressing support showed a decline in market share.

Table 5–3 Letter Responses to HHS from Transplant Centers, 1998

	Oppose rule	No opinion on rule	Support rule	Total
Oppose greater role	30	18	0	48
No opinion on role	28	0	2	30
Support greater role	0	2	5	7
Total	58	20	7	85

Source: Author's calculations based on regulatory docket.

Table 5–4   Characteristics of HHS Final Rule Supporters and Opponents

	All transplants 1998[a]	Liver transplants 1998[a]	Change in liver transplants 1990–1998[a]	Change in liver market share 1990–1998[b]
Oppose greater role	136.6	38.9	54.9	0.006
No opinion on role	150.8	51.3	4.4	–0.405
Support greater role	150.9	56.7	8.7	–0.408
No letter sent	54.0	27.0	4.5	0.020
Oppose liver rule	124.8	38.5	17.9	0.227
No opinion on liver rule	161.0	42.0	4.0	–0.454
Support liver rule	239.4	94.9	–39.0	–2.680

Source: Author's calculations.

[a] Mean.
[b] Percentage points; total market share in percentage points for group in 1998 minus total market share in percentage points for group in 1990.

The picture is clearer with respect to the characteristics of centers conditional on their opinions on national liver allocation. As the last row shows, transplant centers as a group that supported national allocation had suffered declines both in the average number of liver transplants performed, minus 39.0, and in their aggregate market share, minus 2.68 percentage points, from 1990 to 1998. The UPMC alone saw a reduction of 317 liver transplants and a market share loss of 14.1 percentage points over this period. In contrast, centers that wrote in opposition showed increases in average number of transplants, 17.9, and aggregate market share, 0.227 percentage points. Centers that did not express an opinion on liver allocation and those that did not submit letters to the docket had figures between these two extremes. Consequently, this gross comparison confirms the commonly expressed beliefs by both proponents and opponents of national allocation that the position of the other side was motivated by the self-interest of centers.

Although the small sample size warrants caution, simple ordered probit models provide statistical tests of the hypothesis that changes in market share affect the position of transplant centers on liver allocation. Table 5–5 displays the estimated coefficients for two independent variables: change in market share from 1990 to 1998 and the number of centers sharing the center's OPO. The coefficient of the first variable provides the basis for estimating the effect of centers' interests, and the coefficient of the second for estimating the effect of the number of centers already sharing livers from their OPO. The more centers, the more likely they will be to support national sharing, either because they are already sharing more widely or because they would anticipate a smaller marginal impact on local procurement efforts. The first column shows estimates of the model treating those centers that did not submit letters to the docket as having no opinion. The statistically

Table 5–5   Models of Opinion on National Liver Allocation

	All transplant centers (n=290)	Transplant centers submitting letter (n=85)
Change in liver market share 1990–1998	−16.3[a] (5.60)	−14.2[a] (5.69)
Number of centers sharing center's OPO	0.038[a] (0.020)	0.047 (0.039)
Cut point 1	−0.397 (0.155)	0.784 (0.281)
Cut point 2	2.27 (0.219)	1.79 (0.328)
Likelihood ratio test (chi-square, 2 d.f.)	12.60[a]	8.16[a]

Source: Author's analysis.
Note: Ordered categories; oppose, no opinion, support. Standard errors in parentheses.

[a] $p < .05$, one tailed-test.

significant negative coefficient for market share change rejects the hypothesis that market share change has no effect in favor of the alternative hypothesis, that centers that lost market share were more likely to support national allocation and that those that gained share are more likely to oppose it. The statistically significant positive coefficient for number of centers sharing the center's OPO rejects the hypothesis of no effect in favor of more centers contributing to greater support for national sharing. The second column of Table 5–5 shows similar results if the sample is restricted to those centers that submitted letters to the docket.

Tables 5.6 and 5.7 convey the substantive impact of market share change on the probabilities of support and opposition. In the model based on all transplant centers, moving from the mean change in market share for supporters of the liver rule (−2.68 percentage points) to the mean change in market shares for opponents (0.227 percentage points), almost doubles the probability of opposing the rule (28.0 versus 14.5 percent) and more than halves the probability of supporting the rule (1.9 versus 5.4 percent). The second model, which limits analysis to those centers submitting letters, shows similarly large substantive effects. These probabilities assume the mean number of centers per OPO, 5.9. The probability ranges in parentheses show the impact of moving one standard deviation above and below this mean. These ranges are also substantively significant. Overall, the statistical evidence supports the proposition that self-interest influenced the position transplant centers took on the issue of the national allocation of livers.

Table 5–6   Effects of Liver Market Share Change, All Transplant Centers

Change	Oppose	No opinion	Support
0.227	28.0 (32.5, 23.9)	70.1 (66.2, 73.6)	1.9 (1.4, 2.9)
−2.680	14.5 (17.6, 11.8)	80.1 (78.2, 81.2)	5.4 (4.1, 7.0)

Source: Author's calculation.
Note: Probabilities in percentages for 5.9 centers per OPO; probabilities for 2.5 and 9.3 centers per OPO in parentheses.

What arguments were offered in favor of the opinions expressed on a greater role of HHS and the national allocation of livers? Table 5–8 displays the frequencies of various arguments appearing in the eighty-five letters submitted to the docket. Consider the arguments against national allocation in terms of impacts on patients and centers. Several are distributional: a national list will discriminate against low-income and minority populations; new rules will negatively affect small- and medium-sized transplant centers; rules benefit only large transplant centers. Several others are efficiency based: allocating organs to the sickest first increases losses of organs and patient lives; a national system is more costly for the entire transplant community. Interestingly, the most frequently cited argument was related to the impact of national sharing on organ procurement: successful procurement depends on dedication and motivation of local transplant professionals. On the one hand, supporting this argument empirically is difficult, despite its plausibility to transplant surgeons who expend the extra efforts, such as travel within their OPOs, to make the marginal procurement. On the other hand, it resonates with the widely accepted argument that obtaining more organs should be a priority for the transplant community, and the argument by opponents that efforts challenging the existing system would be better invested in developing policies to increase procurement.

Table 5–7   Effects of Liver Market Share Change, Centers Submitting Letters

Change	Oppose	No opinion	Support
0.227	70.5 (75.7, 64.7)	23.4 (19.8, 27.0)	6.1 (4.4, 8.3)
−2.680	54.9 (61.2, 48.5)	32.2 (29.0, 34.9)	12.9 (9.8, 16.6)

Source: Author's calculation.
Note: Probabilities in percentages for 5.9 centers per OPO; probabilities for 2.5 and 9.3 centers per OPO in parentheses.

Table 5–8   Reasons For and Against HHS Rules in 1998 Letters

Supporting greater role	Frequency
Current system lacks self-regulation, equity, and cooperation	1
Government can provide needed oversight while allowing professionals to make medical choices	2
OPTN should be reorganized with less physician-dominance	1
No specific reason; other reasons	2
Opposing greater role	
Government involvement could cause politicization	3
Transplantation decisions should be made physicians and the transplant community	16
UNOS is best equipped to make allocation decisions	12
Government's role is to provide oversight, not to form policy	5
Current system works well	4
No specific reason; other reasons	1
Supporting liver rule	
Organs should be allocated to the most critically ill patients who benefit most	3
Rules provide geographic equity	5
Local medical communities are not focusing on patient needs under current system	1
Patients should have choice of transplant centers based on outcomes and care as well as location	1
Opposing liver rule	
Resources better spent promoting donation, not nationalizing distribution	18
Current system is equitable and scientific	5
Successful procurement depends on dedication and motivation of local transplant professionals	27
A national system would increase waiting lists for livers	7
A national system is more costly for the entire transplant community	16
New rules negatively impact small- and medium-sized transplant centers	26
Mortality rates will increase if new rules take effect	3
Allocating organs to the sickest first increases losses of organs and patient lives	17
Rules only benefit large transplant centers	8
Increases in organ preservation times will negatively affect transplant outcomes	9
National list would discriminate against low-income and minority populations	19
No specific reason	3
Other	6

Source: Author's compilation based on review of regulatory docket following proposed rulemaking (HHS 1994).

State Challenges to National Allocation

The members of transplant communities in a number of states, facing a possible loss of organs, sought to block the effect of the new rule by seeking legislation to keep organs procured within their states for use by transplant centers within the state. A number of states responded to these efforts, both out of concern for state residents on the waiting list and at the urging of transplant centers that feared losses of organs. The common form of the law prohibited export of organs to states with which the state did not have a reciprocal agreement. Such laws were adopted in 1998 and 1999 by Florida, Louisiana, Oklahoma, South Carolina, Tennessee, and Wisconsin. Several other states, including Arizona, Nevada, New Mexico, Ohio, and Texas, adopted resolutions urging Congress to block implementation of the Final Rule.

The effort in Wisconsin was enthusiastically supported by its governor, Tommy Thompson, who had been an advocate over the years for policies to increase organ donation in the state. Wisconsin enjoyed a high donation rate relative to Illinois, which, along with Minnesota, South Dakota, and North Dakota, comprise OPTN Region 7. Wisconsin quickly established reciprocal agreements with Minnesota, South Dakota, and North Dakota. Transplant centers in these states and Wisconsin feared a large outflow of livers to Illinois under regional sharing. Eventually a threat to seek a new region that would exclude Illinois encouraged the Chicago transplant centers to agree to provisions that prevented any transplant center from consistently gaining from the arrangement by requiring all the regionally shared organs be paid back in kind (Marchione 1999).

Wisconsin and Louisiana also challenged the legal authority for the Final Rule in federal court. The Louisiana challenge, *Louisiana v. Shalala*, No. 98-802-C-3m (M.D. La. 1998), resulted in a stay of the Final Rule on September 30, 1998, the day before it was to become effective. The judge subsequently dismissed the HHS appeal to remove the injunction, but did allow the UPMC to join the lawsuit in favor of implementation (McMullen 1999, 408). The following month the case was administratively closed, allowing either party to reopen without prejudice. The Wisconsin suit attempted to block implementation of the revised Final Rule published in October 1999 (HHS 1999), but was dismissed on the grounds that the plaintiffs lacked standing (Grantham 2001, 764). When Thompson became the new secretary of the HHS in the Bush administration, the new governor, Scott McCallum, decided not to appeal the negative decision of the U.S. District Court in November 2000, avoiding the prospect of *Thompson v. Thompson*.

Expanding the liver allocation controversy from the OPTN to the traditional regulatory arena activated a variety of political processes—state lawmaking within federalism to protect local interests, legal challenges seeking judicial review of rulemaking, and, most consequentially, congressional intervention.

Congressional Intervention: Moratorium on Implementation

Meanwhile, Congress had already postponed implementation of the Final Rule from July 1 to October 1, 1998, in an amendment to a spending bill (Public Law 105-174). Members of Congress lined up on both sides of the issue, largely depending on the positions of transplant centers in their states. It is probably safe to say that most members believed that decisions about transplant allocation should be made primarily by medical professionals, although this general belief could translate in very different positions on the appropriate oversight role for HHS.

In June 1998 Sen. Robert Torricelli (D–NJ) introduced a rider to the fiscal-year 1999 appropriations bill for HHS, placing a one-year moratorium on implementation of the Final Rule and calling for a study of various aspects of OPTN policy by the Institute of Medicine of the National Academies. During the debate over the moratorium, several congressional hearings were held on the Final Rule. The political battle under way between UNOS and HHS is evident in the unusually strident comments of Secretary Shalala, made first in prepared testimony to a joint meeting of the Subcommittee on Health and the Environment of the House Commerce Committee and the Senate Labor and Human Resources Committee on June 18, 1998, and repeated verbatim in prepared testimony to the Labor, Health and Human Services, and Education Subcommittee of the Senate Appropriations Committee on September 10, 1998:

> Unfortunately, to this point, UNOS has failed to seize the opportunity offered by the rule to develop consensus about policy improvements. In fact, UNOS has gone to great lengths to preserve the current unfair system. It has launched a cynical political lobbying campaign against the April 2 rule. This campaign has been characterized by misinformation and outright falsehoods. The essence of the UNOS campaign has been to create phantom policies and use scare tactics that have hospital administrators and patients around the country up in arms. UNOS has sent form letters, part of a self-described "legislative action kit," to surgeons and patients across the country. UNOS has been loud and vociferous in its lobbying and is working with some of the highest priced public relations and lobbying firms in town. As a result of their slick lobbying campaign, you are hearing protests about the April 2 rule.

Despite opposition from the Clinton administration, the rider remained part of the final bill that became law in October 1998 (Public Law 105-277).

In February 1999 the Institute of Medicine (IOM) assembled a committee of sixteen medical researchers and clinicians, though no active liver transplant surgeons were included, to answer the questions on organ procurement and transplantation Congress posed. The Committee on Organ Procurement and Transplantation issued its report in July (IOM 1999). The report addressed the full range of issues Congress raised, but invested most of its analytical effort in assessing liver allocation. It presented two empirical findings that strongly undercut the case for fully national sharing. First, waiting times for status 1 and 2A patients (status 1 in table 5–1) did not vary much geographically. Most of the variation in waiting times occurred for status 2B and status 3 patients. In other words, the patients with the most medically urgent conditions in different regions saw similar waiting times so that the major consequence of broader sharing would be reductions in waiting time differences for patients in the less medically urgent categories. Second, based on a review of published studies, the committee concluded that the "medically acceptable cold ischemic time" for livers is twelve hours (IOM 1999, 11) as opposed to the twelve to eighteen hours cited in the Final Rule notice (HHS 1998a, 16304), suggesting that regional rather than national sharing was more consistent with the scientific evidence on organ viability. Therefore, rather than endorse national allocation of livers, the committee recommended that the areas for local allocation comprise populations of at least 9 million people, a population larger than that served by most OPOs but smaller than that of OTPN regions. Recognizing the importance of relationships that have evolved among OPOs and transplant centers, however, the committee recommended that these larger areas be formed through sharing arrangements among existing OPOs. The revised Final Rule published on October 20, 1999, reflected the findings of the IOM report. In particular, it dropped use of the controversial term national list and "directs the OPTN to overcome as much as possible arbitrary geographic barriers" (HHS 1999, 56651).

Despite the softening on national allocation, there remained considerable opposition in Congress to the increased HHS role in allocation policy. Rep. Michael Bilirakis (R–FL) introduced a bill (H 2418) to overturn the HHS Final Rule, stating in the floor debate that medical experts "and not Secretary Shalala know best when it comes to transplant policy" (Carey 2000, 838). HR 2418, as amended, nullified the rule and prevented HHS from asserting final authority over allocation policies. On April 4, 2000, it passed the House 275 to 147, with Republicans supporting it 187 to 26 and Democrats opposing it 120 to 87.

Was support or opposition by members of the House based on party, ideology, or the interests of transplant centers in their districts? It would be surprising if representatives were not influenced by the positions of the centers in their districts, especially on an issue for which the personnel of the centers would likely be the most vocal and credible voices they heard. At the same time, one might expect that, other things equal, Democrats would be more likely to vote against HR 2418 in support of the administration. The more interesting question, however, is whether or not ideology had an effect. Conservatives might support nullification of the rule as blocking undesirable federal interference in medical affairs; liberals might oppose nullification out of an egalitarian concern about disparities across regions.

To investigate the sources of support for HR 2418, table 5–9 presents probit models of its roll call. Model 1 includes the member's party (1 for Democrats, 0 otherwise), ideology as measured by the Americans for Democratic Action (ADA) score (0 to 100, with 100 most liberal), whether the member's district included a transplant center that submitted a letter to the regulatory docket in opposition to the HHS rule (1 if yes, 0 otherwise), or whether the member's district included a transplant center that submitted a letter to the regulatory docket in support of the HHS rule (1 if yes, 0 otherwise). The positions of transplant centers in the district have statistically significant effects as predicted. Ideology has a statistically significant effect on the probability of supporting the bill, but party does not: more liberal members were less likely to vote yes, but Democrats were not. Overall, the model correctly predicts 77 percent of the cases with roughly symmetric errors in contrast to the 65 percent that would be correctly classified if all cases were predicted to be in the modal yes category. Model 2 shows stable results when party is removed from the model.

As ideology and party are highly correlated (0.91), it is worth checking to see whether multicollinearity is suppressing the effect of party. Indeed, model 3, which removes

Table 5–9   Roll Call Analysis of HR 2418

Variable	Model 1	Model 2	Model 3
Party, 1 Democrat, 0 other	.15 (.33)		−1.4[a] (.14)
Americans for Democratic Action score	−2.4[a] (.45)	−2.2[a] (.21)	
Center in district opposes HHS	.65[a] (.20)	.64[a] (.20)	.43[a] (.19)
Center in district supports HHS	−1.9[a] (.74)	−1.9[a] (.74)	−1.9[a] (.68)
Constant	1.4[a] (.13)	1.4[a] (.13)	1.1[a] (.11)
Observations[b]	421	421	422
Likelihood ratio test (chi-square, 4 or 3 d. f.)	143.9[a]	143.7[a]	115.4[a]
Correct predictions	.77	.77	.75

Source: Author's compilation.
Probit model: 1 for, 0 against; standard errors in parentheses.

[a] $p < .05$
[b] Vote was 275 for; 147 against. ADA score missing for one member.

ideology, does show a statistically significant effect for party, and prevents us from completely ruling out party as an influence on the vote. Nevertheless, the statistically significant coefficient for ideology and the statistically insignificant coefficient for party in model 1 somewhat favor ideology as an explanation.

In the other chamber, Sen. Bill Frist (R–TN), himself a transplant surgeon, introduced a bill (S 2366) to create a board of medical experts and patients to establish allocation policy. As part of a compromise with Sen. Ted Kennedy (D–MA) and Secretary Shalala, Frist agreed to amendments that would give the Secretary a greater role in determining the composition of the board. Although the compromise version was approved 18 to 0 by the Health, Education, Labor and Pensions Committee, Sen. Russ Feingold (D–WI) prevented it from being voted on in the Senate before the spring recess at the urging of the Coalition of Major Transplant Centers, a group of twenty hospitals organized by a Wisconsin transplant surgeon. The coalition argued that the compromise bill would give HHS too large a role in allocation policy. With the anticipated difficulty of resolving the large differences between the House and Senate bills in conference committee, and the promised veto of any bill similar to the House version by President Clinton, the 106th Congress ended without legislation on organ allocation.

Denouement: Convergence of OPTN and HHS Positions on Liver Allocation

Throughout the period of regulatory and legislative conflict, various OPTN committees continued their ongoing efforts to improve the liver allocation system. These efforts resulted in a number of changes in OPTN policy: establishing voluntary guidelines for patient listing criteria in 1996; establishing regional review boards (RRBs) for retrospective reviews of status assignments; removing chronic patients from status 1 as previously discussed; introducing separate medical urgency criteria for pediatric patients in1997; introducing a more objective scoring system for assessing severity of liver disease for non–status 1 patients in 1998; establishing priority of regional status 1 patients over non–status 1 local patients in 1999; and establishing a separate pediatric scoring system in 2000. (The separate pediatric allocation system was based on evidence that pediatric livers produce larger gains in survival rates for pediatric patients than for adult patients.)

The introduction of the RRBs was an important preliminary step for sharing beyond local areas. Recall that abandoning the UNOS/STAT designation in 1991 was due in no small part to concerns that some transplant centers were gaming the system by inappropriately classifying patients to obtain livers under the emergency designation. Particular concerns about such behavior at three Chicago-area hospitals were later verified in the context of a fraudulent billing suit filed by the federal government revealing that during the 1990s liver patients listed as critically ill were actually not in the hospital (Murphy 2004). Centers would be reluctant to participate in wider sharing unless they believed that there was compliance with classification criteria. The RRBs include representatives from all liver transplant centers in the region. They conduct retrospective reviews of all status 1 cases. In addition, they handle prospective requests for special treatment of exceptional cases under the severity rating system. If the RRB does not respond within twenty-one days, then the center may list the patient at the requested score. The RRB refers cases involving inappropriate classifications, or cases it is unable to resolve, to the Liver and Intestinal Organ Transplantation Committee for review. Centers found by the committee to be inappropriately classifying patients may be referred to the Membership and Professional Standards Committee for disciplinary action. For example, at meetings in January, May, July, and October 2001, the committee reviewed twenty cases, overturning an RRB in one case, resolving two cases the RRBs could not, and supporting them in the remaining cases. The committee voted to refer centers with multiple violations to the Membership and Professional Standards Committee.

The new liver allocation system uses the severity formula developed in the model for end-stage liver disease (MELD). Initiated by researchers at the Mayo Clinic, MELD was designed to predict the probability of mortality within three months for liver patients (Forman and Lucy 2001; Kamath et al. 2001). It provides an alternative to the older Pugh-Child-Turcotte classification of medical urgency. It also offers a ranking criterion to replace waiting time as a factor in liver allocation, as recommended by the Institute of Medicine study. A pediatric version, pediatric end-stage liver disease (PELD), was also developed. A number of adjustments to the rating systems were made as they became part of the proposed new liver allocation rules.

The process that produced these changes involved interaction among a number of OPTN committees, particularly the Liver Disease Severity Scale Committee, the Liver and

Intestinal Organ Transplantation Committee, the Liver Distribution Unit Committee, and the Pediatric Transplantation Committee. It involved the seeking of comments from interested parties and the public, and a public forum on liver allocation held in Dallas, Texas, on September 28, 2000. The process is also viewed by the participants as ongoing. As noted in a UNOS briefing paper describing the changes, "the concept envisioned by the Committees is one that allows continuous quality improvement of the organ allocation policy, one that can and should be regularly modified in a timely manner as more data and experience is [sic] gained" (2002a, 3). For example, pointing to the MELD and PELD scoring systems based on pre-transplant mortality risk, the "logical next step" is to develop models for predicting mortality among patients who receive transplants (4).

The Distribution Units Committee considered alternative ways to define local and regional units, but did not have data available to assess fully other than population as a basis for distribution units. Using a patient-based simulation model for its analysis, the committee concluded that there were no clear advantages from redefining distribution units to achieve the minimum population size of 9 million people the Institute of Medicine recommended (Harper et al. 2000; Freeman, Harper, and Edwards 2002). Further, the committee judged it prudent to await implementation of MELD scores, which would likely have a substantial impact in directing organs to patients most in need. It therefore recommended that, rather than redefine distribution units, regions should be encouraged to develop broader sharing mechanisms. The board of directors accepted the recommendation in November 2000.

The basic outline of the proposed liver allocation system shown in table 5–10 was approved by the Liver and Intestinal Organ Transplantation Committee in October 2001 and by the board of directors the following month. Additional changes were approved by the Executive Committee on February 1, 2002 and were incorporated into the OPTN policies in June 2002.

The new liver allocation rules show substantial movement toward broader geographic sharing—particularly with respect to giving regional status 1 patients priority over local patients who were not status 1. Because the rules appear consistent with the revised Final Rule that HHS adopted, it was not rejected by the board established in the revised Final Rule to advise the secretary on OPTN policy, and therefore not rejected by the secretary. Further, the liver allocation rules as implemented by the OPTN have continued to evolve.

Implementation of regional sharing shows the adaptive and incremental nature of decision making in the OPTN. Procedures exist for local and regional modifications of allocation rules under UNOS Policy 3.4.6. Alternative allocation units, typically grouping OPOs for local allocation, may be formed and provisionally approved for three years if they are deemed to correct an inequity in allocation; evidence of improvement in terms of meeting objective criteria must be provided for continuation after the probationary period. As discussed in chapter 3, variances to point systems used in allocation and the formation of alternative sharing arrangements among OPOs may also be proposed and approved. These mechanisms have allowed for considerable experimentation in allocation.

In the case of liver allocation, Region 1 (New England) has played a key role. It began an alternative sharing arrangement in 1990, and formalized it in 1995, to allocate available organs to status 1 patients on a regional basis (Rohrer 1996). In 1999 Region 1 obtained a variance to replace the liver allocation rules then in place with a point scale

Table 5–10   Allocation of Adult Livers to Adult Patients, 2002

Patient status
Status 1. Fulminant liver failure with life expectancy of less than seven days. Status 1 patients revert to most recent model for end-stage liver disease (MELD) score after seven days.
All other patients with MELD scores greater than 6.
All other patients with MELD scores equal to 6 (minimum possible score) placed on common list with pediatric patients with a pediatric end-stage liver disease (PELD) score of less than or equal to 6.

Geographic-status priority
1. Local status 1 patients in descending point order
2. Regional status 1 patients in descending point order
3. All other local patients in descending point order
4. All other regional patients in descending point order
5. National status 1 patients in descending point order
6. All other national patients in descending point order

Priority
MELD score based on measures of creatinine, bilirubin, prothrombin time (INR), and disease etiology used to estimate risk of mortality while on transplant waiting list.
Current MELD score formula (maximum 40):
$10 [0.957 \ln(\text{creatinine mg/dL}) + 0.378 \ln(\text{milirubin mg/dL}) + 1.120 \ln(\text{INR}) + 0.643]$
Allocation based on rounded MELD score. Priority among patients with same MELD score determined by waiting time at that score.

Source: Author's compilation based on UNOS 2002a.

that de-emphasized waiting time and used a continuous medical urgency scale to prioritize allocation among status 2B patients (Freeman et al. 2001). It thus demonstrated the feasibility of the two major components of the current liver allocation system: regional sharing for status 1 patients and priority based on a continuous scale of medical need for other patients.

In approving regional sharing of livers for status 1 patients in June 1999, the board of directors instructed the Liver and Intestinal Organ Committee to work with regions to develop alternative sharing arrangements that would take advantage of regional experience and allay regional concerns. This process led to a variety of alternative sharing arrangements. Several regions adopted the standard allocation system with no, or only minor, changes. Regions 2 (Mid-Atlantic), 4 (Texas and Oklahoma), 5 (California and Southwest), 7 (Upper Midwest), and 8 (Central), however, initially modified regional sharing to include payback provisions to ensure that regional allocation does not consistently favor transplant centers in any particular OPO. For example, reflecting tensions between Wisconsin and Illinois transplant centers, the Region 7 arrangement required, with some exceptions, that the OPO receiving a regionally allocated liver provide the next liver it procures of the same blood type to the donor OPO; by contrast, Region 4 required payback only when a debt of three livers had accumulated. Interestingly, such payback provisions are similar to the rota used to equalize allocation among liver transplant centers in the United Kingdom (UK Transplant 1999).

Noting that under the Final Rule variances to allocation rules should be limited to local experiments that could be used to influence nationwide rules, the Liver and Intestinal Organ Transplantation Committee recommended that the regions be required to reassess the necessity of their payback arrangements in light of the improved patient classification system that reduces the opportunity for gaming the waiting list. (All but Region 2 had adopted the payback arrangements before the MELD standardization and related changes to the patient classification system that substantially reduced opportunities for gaming.) The board of directors voted to eliminate payback provisions at its November 2005 meeting.

The implementation of the new sharing agreement also shows how the bottom-up process can change general policies. Under the rules in place in 1999, a request for an alternative sharing arrangement required unanimous support by all the OPOs and transplant centers involved. Region 5 was unable to obtain unanimity for its proposal. The committee responded by recommending to the board that the threshold for consideration of proposals be lowered to 75 percent agreement, which the board voted to accept in November 2000.

The regional agreements demonstrated the feasibility of regional sharing of livers for the sickest patients. At its June 2004 meeting, the board of directors generalized regional sharing by amending liver allocation policies to give priority to patients with MELD or PELD scores of fifteen or higher within the region over less medically urgent local patients with lower scores.

Would the rules have evolved as quickly and substantially as they have without the HHS rulemaking? Of course, the argument that the rules would have remained approximately as they were in the mid-1990s had they not become a focus of the rulemaking cannot be ruled out with absolute certainty—even though HHS itself saw changes in OPTN liver allocation policies before 1996, including UNOS/STAT, as representing "attempts to favor the most urgent needs" (HHS 1998a, 16318). It should be kept in mind, however, that it was OPTN revisions of the liver allocation rules that provided the impetus for revival of the rulemaking in 1996. More generally, the continual reassessment of policies by the OPTN committees suggests that considerable change in the liver allocation rules would have occurred, perhaps less quickly, even in the absence of the Final Rule.

A major impact of the controversy was almost certainly greater pressure on the OPTN to strengthen the scientific basis for its rulemaking. As the chair of the Liver and Intestinal Organ Transplantation Committee during the latter part of the controversy reflected, "I think the debate in 96-97 stimulated all of us to better define the variables and provide better justification for the policies we were advocating; in effect, to make us prove that we were 'more expert' than the public rule makers" (Richard Freeman, personal communication to the author, August 12, 2003). Staff of the HHS Office of Transplantation see the awarding of separate contracts for the administration of the OPTN and the Scientific Registry of Transplant Recipients (SRTR) as facilitating independent empirical investigations in support of policy development (Richard Durbin, interview with the author, September 20, 2002). A number of day-long committee meetings attended by the author over the last seven years consistently showed extensive use of evidence, including reports from the SRTR staff, reports by independent researchers, data assembled by UNOS staff, and information brought to the table by committee members. Chapters 6 and 7 consider these processes in more detail in the context of the evolution of kidney allocation rules.

Conclusion

What does the controversy over the Final Rule and liver allocation tell us about the advantages and disadvantages of the OPTN as a form of private rulemaking and as a potential model for medical governance?

First, the continuous involvement of the OPTN in issues through its standing committees allows for the sort of evolutionary change that Ross Cheit found in his comparison of public and private standard-setting (1990). In the controversy over liver allocation, there were two sources of change: the internal dynamics of the members of the network and the oversight by HHS. One can point to other important areas of policy where the internal dynamic has dominated. For example, as discussed in chapter 6, the OPTN made a number of incremental changes to the kidney allocation system in response to concerns about its consequences for racial disparities in waiting time. More recently, one can also identify cases in which HHS has played a role in speeding up change as in prompting the OPTN to begin to set standards for live donations as discussed in chapter 4. Further, the potential for HHS to reject rules has reinforced the continued move toward fully regional sharing of livers for the sickest patients.

The internal dynamic leading to evolutionary change depends on binding votes—a majority of the board of directors can change OPTN policies. One advantage of voting is that it can be easily applied to specific elements of any particular proposal for change. Another is that it allows change in the absence of a consensus. Of course, this may also be a disadvantage if the distribution of votes does not match well the distribution of interests. As shown in the Final Rule controversy, for example, the UPMC was not able to achieve broader geographic sharing as quickly as it had hoped, despite its prominent role as a transplant center, leading it to seek change through public rulemaking where its prominence and size gave it a relatively more influential voice. This challenge to the network moved debate dramatically into the political sphere, prompting efforts by states and Congress to protect threatened interests.

The internal dynamic is also facilitated by the use of variances by the OPTN. For example, the variance implemented by Region 1 to allocate livers regionally experimented with a prerequisite of wider allocation, more confident ranking of patients in terms of medical need, and demonstrated its feasibility; the allowance for payback provisions eased concerns about gaming within several of the regions during implementation of regional sharing until the various changes intended to reduce opportunism were shown to be effective. HHS could also allow for variances as it did in the area of state welfare policies leading up to welfare reform, but the process would likely be less flexible because of the value of uniformity in national policy under public rulemaking. The advantage of experimentation through variances is the opportunity to develop an empirical basis for assessing potential policy change. The disadvantage is that it results in different treatment of similar patients in different locales.

Looking to the possible use of private rulemaking in other contexts, it is important to note that the OPTN itself represents an evolutionary change, that it has a well-defined substantive focus, and that stakeholder interests tend to align with patient interests. Voluntary sharing by UNOS was already under way when the OPTN was created, so that its members had considerable experience with cooperating as well as plausible starting points from which allocation policy could begin to evolve. In the absence of such experience, implementing private rulemaking would likely be more difficult. The evolutionary nature of private rulemaking would also place great importance on the initial policies chosen, an uncertain task in the absence of previous cooperation. Although the technology of organ transplantation is highly complex, the OPTN responsibility for developing procurement and allocation policies gives rulemaking a clear focus. Appropriately applying private rulemaking in other contexts would require drawing boundaries broad enough so important trade-offs are considered, but not so broadly as to invite shifting issues to the larger political arena. Within the context of allocation, the interests of transplant surgeons are aligned closely to those of at least their own patients. The absence of such alignment would require more aggressive oversight to prevent the private rulemaker from acting primarily as a stakeholder cartel.

Second, the OPTN shows the effective continuous engagement of expertise in rulemaking. OPTN committees have a heavy representation of transplant surgeons who bring the sort of tacit knowledge—information and understanding based on firsthand experience and observation—that is extremely useful in identifying potential issues to be addressed as well as in predicting the likely consequences of proposed rule changes. Many of these surgeons also contribute to the medical literature on transplantation, which gives them considerable experience in dealing with empirical evidence. Further, the OPTN committees closely connect expertise to policy questions, a feature observers see as a characteristic of the most effective federal advisory panels (Jasanoff 1990, 230–31; Bruce L.R. Smith 1992, 193).

One can imagine HHS using similar committees as expert panels to support public rulemaking for organ procurement and allocation. The ethos of the advisory committee would likely be for members to avoid conflicts of interest in giving advice. To the extent interests were removed from advice, the politics of rulemaking would likely appear in connection with publication of proposed rulemakings rather than within the committee. One consequence is that the stakeholders would not be able to shape as confidently the detailed content of rules because any compromises made within the committee could be undone when the agency drafted the rule. Indeed, anticipating the possibility of challenging the agency rule in court might lead stakeholders to be less than forthcoming with their tacit knowledge—this is one of the concerns that negotiated rulemaking is intended to address, though on an episodic rather than ongoing basis. Transplant surgeons would probably be less willing to participate in advisory panels than in OPTN committees. Also, they would likely form organizations to represent their particular interests in public rulemaking as well as in the legislative process that oversees it.

Before accepting this preliminary assessment of the OPTN as an attractive form of medical governance, especially for complex problems where tacit knowledge is essential, it is important to assess more than one case. The next two chapters consider OPTN rulemaking with respect to kidney allocation.

6

Incremental Response to Racial Disparity in Kidney Allocation

Good public policy strikes a reasoned balance among valid but usually competing social goals. Allocating transplant kidneys to maximize the chances that recipients survive is certainly desirable. Allocating them equitably is desirable as well. Yet these goals may conflict in a variety of ways. Most prominently, medical efficacy and equity of access have come into conflict over decisions about how much weight to place on antigen matching between deceased donors and kidney transplant recipients in allocation rules. Although antigen matching increases graft and transplant survival rates, it reduces the opportunities for African Americans to receive timely transplants. The responses of the OPTN to this conflict of goals further reveal the nature of incremental change through private rulemaking.

Patterns of kidney transplantation starkly differ by race. People identifying as African American or black comprise only about 13 percent of the U.S. population. Nonetheless, at the beginning of 2008 African Americans accounted for almost 35 percent of people on the waiting list for kidney transplants—more than twenty-seven thousand compared to about thirty-one thousand whites. The median waiting times for blacks and whites who joined the waiting list in 2001 and 2002 were 1,849 and 1,283 days, respectively, a difference of more than eighteen months. For this same cohort, the percentages of blacks and whites receiving transplants within one year (two years) were 10.1 (20.5) and 16.2 (30.8), respectively. In 2007, 7,630 whites and 3,427 blacks received kidney transplants and 1,729 whites and 1,113 blacks were removed from the waiting list because they had died. For those receiving kidney transplants over the seven years ending in 2004, the one-year (five-year) survival rates for blacks and whites were 88.9 (60.8) percent and 92.1 (73.9) percent, respectively (OPTN 2009). Thus, on average, blacks wait longer for transplants and experience less successful outcomes than whites.

One explanation for the racial imbalance of the kidney transplant waiting list is the higher prevalence of end-stage renal disease (ESRD) among blacks than whites. Approximately 32 percent of the 485,000 people with ESRD in 2005 were black (USRDS 2008, table B.1). Longer waiting times, however, also result from the rules that guide allocation. Specifically, the use of antigen matching disadvantages blacks on the waiting list. Antigen patterns correlate with race, so that with disproportionate numbers on the waiting list and only roughly proportional kidney donation rates (14.8 percent of deceased and 11.7

percent of living donors in 2008 were African American), the opportunity for matches is lower for blacks than for whites.

A number of factors contribute to the lower survival rates for blacks relative to whites. Blacks are less likely to receive living-donor transplants, which have higher success rates than deceased-donor transplants. Longer waits to receive transplants, perhaps exacerbated by delays in joining the list following the onset of ESRD, result in poorer health, which in turn reduces survival rates. Fairness in access to timely transplants literally has life and death implications.

To assess how the OPTN has addressed controversy over racial disparity in kidney allocation, this chapter begins with a brief history of dialysis and kidney transplantation. It next looks specifically at the issue of racial disparity in kidney allocation. Finally, it considers several incremental changes to national allocation rules made by the OPTN in response to racial disparity. These changes show the capacity of OPTN governance to assess scientific information and tacit knowledge in responding to value conflicts.

Dialysis and Kidney Transplantation

The evolution of kidney transplantation policy was influenced in several ways by the introduction of the artificial kidney, or dialysis, as a clinical treatment in the 1960s. First, as noted in chapter 3, the federal government responded to limited access to dialysis with the ESRD program in 1972. Efforts to control the costs of this program led to federal investments that encouraged kidney transplantation and the growth of the voluntary network of transplant centers. Second, the proliferation of dialysis centers in response to federal coverage through the ESRD program allowed more patients to survive for longer periods without transplants. One consequence is an increase in the number of people waiting at any time for a transplant. Another consequence, potentially relevant to racial disparity, is that dialysis centers do not have a strong incentive to list patients for transplants, and thus less proactive patients may not be listed, or may be listed later, than their more proactive counterparts. Third, and most relevant to kidney allocation, the use of social values in allocating the initially very limited supply of dialysis treatment by several centers set the stage for more formal, and defensible, allocation rules in kidney transplantation.

The Artificial Kidney and Social Allocation

An artificial kidney, or hemodialyzer, can keep ESRD patients alive by filtering toxic wastes from the blood that would normally be removed by a functioning kidney. Although used on an experimental basis for humans since the 1940s, dialysis was impractical for long-term maintenance treatment because repeated use would eventually exhaust body sites suitable for connecting the machine to blood vessels. The introduction in 1960 of an indwelling cannula (small tube), a device that could be surgically implanted to permit repeated attachment of the machine over an indefinite period, made dialysis practical for long-term maintenance of patients with ESRD. Although later peritoneal dialysis, which involves the cycling of fluid into and out of the belly to absorb impurities from the blood, gave ESRD patients a choice of treatment mode, initially hemodialysis provided through centers, either on-site or at home, was the only option.

Detailed and insightful accounts of the initial years of dialysis and the origins of the Medicare ESRD entitlement provided by Richard Rettig (1982, 1991) are the main sources for the following brief overview.

The first dialysis center was established in 1962 by Dr. Belding Scribner, who developed the indwelling cannula that permitted repeated connection to the dialysis machine. The Seattle Artificial Kidney Center immediately faced more demand for dialysis than it could supply, forcing it to allocate available openings among patients. Those who received dialysis had their lives extended; those who did not typically died within a short time. The center followed a two-stage allocation process that later became highly controversial. The first stage involved screening by physicians on the Medical Advisory Committee, which applied criteria to determine medical suitability. In addition to applying clear clinical criteria, such as level of renal function and absence of certain then-relevant contraindications, the committee limited selection to stable and emotionally mature adults under forty-five years old with a demonstrated willingness to carry out the treatment regime, including dietary restrictions. In the second stage, medically suitable candidates were referred to the Admissions and Policy Committee, an anonymous group initially consisting of a lawyer, minister, housewife, labor leader, state government official, banker, surgeon, and two physicians who served as advisors (Fox and Swazey 1974, 244). As described in an exposé in *Life* magazine by Shana Alexander in 1962, the committee did not apply formal criteria, but rather considered on a case-by-case basis such social factors as number of dependents, potential service to society, character, and moral strength. Other early artificial kidney centers dealt with the allocation problem in different ways. For example, the Cleveland Clinic used a first-come, first-served criterion, possibly explaining its lower initial success rate in keeping patients alive. Physicians at Peter Bent Brigham Hospital in Boston integrated social criteria into their clinical decision making. Overall, a majority of dialysis centers used some sort of social value criteria in their allocation decisions (Kilner 1990, 28).

The negative publicity artificial kidney centers received for delegating the responsibility for selection of dialysis recipients to lay committees that used social criteria had two important consequences. Most immediately, the centers abandoned lay selection committees and replaced them with professional staffs trained in social work, psychology, or nursing (Dennis 1995, 97). The nephrologists who ran the centers, as well as transplant surgeons, "were pulled by conflicting impulses: first, to use fine-grained criteria in order to optimize the amount of well-being from each treatment and second, to find nondiscretionary selection methods that could purchase social acceptance and peace of mind" (Dennis 1995, 99). The second impulse began to dominate as physicians abandoned explicit application of social criteria and sought more formal allocation rules based on medical suitability.

The longer term consequence was to set the stage for federal involvement that would eliminate the scarcity that dictated dialysis rationing. The initial moves were by the Department of Veterans Affairs, which in 1963 proposed to open dialysis centers in a number of its hospitals, and the Public Health Service, which created a grant program in 1965 to support dialysis demonstrations. Anticipating the possibility of increasing federal budgetary outlays to support dialysis through these early programs, in 1966 the Bureau of the Budget convened a committee of experts, the Committee on Chronic Kidney Disease, to advise it on treatment of ESRD. The committee, commonly referred to by the surname of its chair, Carl Gottshalk, concluded in its report that dialysis and transplantation were no longer experimental treatments and recommended creation of a national treatment program through Medicare. The Bureau of the Budget, facing the increasing costs of the Vietnam War, "sought to minimize its impact and its distribution and did nothing to implement its recommendations" (Rettig 1982, 119). It also began trimming the budgets of the Public Health Service programs aimed at demonstrating the feasibility of center- and especially home-based dialysis.

Despite general opposition from the Nixon administration, Congress included support for ESRD patients in a number of programs and pressured Veterans Affairs to open some of its dialysis centers to nonveterans. The patchwork nature of these approaches, however, left many ESRD patients uncovered and introduced uncertainty about the continuation of care through existing programs relying on annual budget appropriations. ESRD patients, their families, and their medical providers increasingly expressed their frustration to members of Congress.

In 1969 the National Kidney Foundation hired a staffer to work full time on lobbying Congress to implement the Gottshalk committee recommendations (Schreiner 2000). Sen. Russell Long (D–LA) became the leading advocate for coverage of ESRD under Medicare. His Senate Finance Committee, as well as the House Ways and Means Committee, held hearings on it. A patient actually underwent dialysis on-site during the second hearing held by the Ways and Means Committee. Ultimately only the Senate bill added the ESRD to Medicare. In the conference committee, Senator Long argued vigorously for another provision, a drug benefit under Medicare. Failing on this major, and very costly, provision, he later argued for the ESRD provision so that the Senate would get something out of the conference, and he prevailed (Plante 2000). The resulting legislation, Public Law 92-603, provided coverage for ESRD as an entitlement to most Americans through section 299I of the Social Security Amendments of 1972. As discussed in chapter 3, the growing cost of the ESRD set the stage for the federal efforts to promote transplantation as a less costly and more desirable alternative to dialysis. By 1991 there were more than two thousand dialysis centers in the United States; by 2005, the number had grown to almost five thousand (USRDS 2007, table J6). By 2005, total Medicare spending on ESRD patients had risen to more than $20 billion, 6.4 percent of the entire Medicare budget (224).

Primary Factors Relevant to Kidney Allocation

Kidneys are far from homogenous goods. Aside from obvious physical attributes such as size and functioning, kidneys differ in other important ways relevant to transplant success. Further, these differences depend not just on the donor kidney but on the biological characteristics of the recipient—an ideal kidney for one recipient may not be a feasible alternative for another.

Three factors are of primary importance in kidney allocation: donor and recipient blood compatibility, human leucocyte antigen (HLA) matching, and recipient sensitization.

Each of these factors has a firm biological basis. Each also has a basis in clinical evidence, although the importance of each has changed over time as other aspects of transplantation technology, especially immunosuppressive drug treatment, have progressed.

Blood Group Compatibility

ABO blood groupings divide people into four blood types: O, A, B, and AB. People with blood type O can donate kidneys to, but not receive kidneys from, the other blood types. In general, good prospects for graft survival require that type A recipients receive kidneys from type A or O donors and type B recipients receive kidneys from type B or O donors. Type AB recipients can receive kidneys from any donors. One important exception to these ABO compatibility rules is that type B recipients can have successful grafts from one of the two major subgroups of type A donors—specifically, type A_2, which accounts for about 15 percent of those with type A. B recipients may also be compatible with A_2B donors. Currently, national allocation rules require that recipients and deceased donors have the standard ABO compatibilities.

Allocation within blood group has consequences for racial disparity in access to kidney transplantation because African Americans are more likely to have type B blood than the general population. As shown in table 6–1, the distribution of blood types of whites on the kidney waiting list closely matches the distribution of blood types of deceased donors. The distribution of blood types among blacks on the list, however, does not closely match the distribution of blood types of donors in general. Compared to the 11.5 percent of deceased donors who are type B, 12.1 percent of whites and 21.4 percent of blacks on the kidney transplant waiting list are type B. Compared to the 35.6 percent of deceased donors who are type A, 35.9 percent of whites and 22.8 percent of blacks on the waiting list are type A. Thus, ignoring the overrepresentation of blacks on the waiting list and allocating kidneys completely randomly within blood groups, blacks have higher odds than whites of receiving a kidney if they are type A but lower odds if they are type B.

Table 6–1   Importance of Blood Type in Kidney Allocation, 2007 (percentages)

Blood type	Deceased donors	Blacks on waiting list	Whites on waiting list	Total on waiting list
O	49.0	52.5	49.2	52.3
A	35.6	22.8	35.9	28.6
B	11.5	21.4	12.1	16.2
AB	3.9	3.3	2.8	2.9

Source: Author's compilation based on OPTN data as of March 17, 2008.

HLA Matching

The first successful transplants were between identical twins who shared the same genetic makeup. As kidney transplantation expanded to include nontwin donors, efforts were made to identify genetic similarity to lessen the recipient's immune reaction that, without some sort of suppression, results in rejection of the graft. Researchers developed the science of histocompatibility to identify the most important genetically determined antigens to better achieve graft success.

Three pairs of antigens, articulated as proteins on cell surfaces, have been identified as particularly relevant to transplantation: HLA-A, HLA-B, and HLA-DR. At each of these three loci, one antigen is inherited from the mother and one from the father—UNOS currently recognizes thirty, sixty-five, and twenty-one distinct antigens at the HLA-A, HLA-B, and HLA-DR loci, respectively (OPTN 2007, appendix 3A). Antigens can be typed as either one of a list of previously identified antigens or as blank. Blanks occur either when both antigens in the pair are the same, so only one antigen is detected at the locus, or when the antigen present has not been identified. Blanks due to unidentified antigens occur disproportionately for members of racial minority groups because they are more likely to have antigens that are rare in the larger population.

Tissue typing involves identifying the antigens present at these loci. Tissue matching involves comparing the number of matches, or more commonly the absence of mismatches, between a specific donor and potential recipient. Because HLA matching considers only a specific set of genetically based antigens, a direct test of the presence of any antigens that would preclude a successful graft, called the crossmatch, is done before the transplant by mixing blood sera of the donor and potential recipient to detect positive reactions. A necessary condition for an acceptable match is a negative crossmatch.

The biological theory underlying HLA matching is firm. However, the clinical importance of the degree of mismatch for graft success has been controversial since its first use in the allocation of cadaveric kidneys (Dennis 1995, 121–26). From the time kidney allocation rules were first established, there has been consensus that either six matches or zero mismatches significantly improves graft success, but considerable disagreement about the extent to which fewer than six matches (or more than zero mismatches) were clinically relevant to graft success. Improvements in immosuppression treatment, which many believe has reduced the importance of HLA matching over time, have complicated the discussion. For example, a recent study found that, for kidney transplants done in 1995, three or more mismatches increased the risk of graft failure relative to zero mismatches, and six mismatches increased relative risk to 1.265, but that, by 1998, only six mismatches showed a statistically significant increase in risk relative to zero mismatches and this increase, 1.152, was smaller than in 1995 (Su et al. 2004).

As with blood types, the frequencies of various antigens differ across races. As cadaveric donation occurs roughly in proportion to racial representation in the population, the majority of donated kidneys, 68 percent in 2007, were from white donors. However, as already noted, blacks comprise 35 percent of the kidney waiting list. Consequently, white patients are much more likely to have close HLA matches to donors than black patients are. Any allocation system that places weight on HLA matching disadvantages blacks relative to whites in terms of access to cadaveric kidneys.

Sensitization

Beyond the genetically based HLA-A, HLA-B, and HLA-DR antigens, dozens of other antigens that develop over one's life course can prevent or reduce the chances of a successful kidney graft. Blood transfusions, pregnancies, and, especially, unsuccessful earlier grafts can produce relevant antigens. Sensitized patients have antigens that preclude them from receiving kidneys from a significant proportion of potential donors. In other words, the more sensitized a patient, the less likely he or she will be an appropriate recipient of the next available cadaveric kidney.

Until recently, the standard technique for assessing sensitivity has been the panel reactive antibody (PRA) test, which exposes the cells of a representative sample of the donor population from the region to serum from the patient. The proportion of donor cells that react are taken as a measure of sensitivity. By convention, if 80 percent or more of the cells react, the patient is considered highly sensitized.

The PRA test has a number of limitations. First, it requires some judgment in setting thresholds for classifying a donor as reactive. Usually, some fraction of each donor's cells react, indicating the strength of the reaction. Histocompatibility laboratories and transplant centers must set specific thresholds for declaring a reaction positive, which leads to some variability in the assessment of the sensitization of transplant patients across centers. Second, the test does not fully indicate the specific sources of the reactions, and therefore does not communicate much information about the likelihood of a negative crossmatch with any particular donor.

More recently, the computed panel reactive antibody (CPRA) method has been introduced to provide a more accurate and informative assessment of sensitivity. It uses the new single-antigen bead assay technology made possible by recombinant DNA procedures. Each bead is sensitive to a single antigen so that its reaction with the patient's blood provides an indication of the presence and strength of that antigen. As with the PRA test, the CPRA method requires laboratories and transplant centers to set thresholds for deciding when an antigen is relevant. Rather than reporting an overall percentage of reactions, the specific patient antigens the transplant center judges as precluding a transplant are listed. Sensitivity is then calculated based on the frequencies of those antigens in the relevant donor population.

The switch to CPRA offers a number of advantages (Geier 2008). First, it contributes to greater uniformity and accountability in determining sensitivity. Listing more antigens increases the calculated sensitization, but also excludes more potential donors from consideration. Transplant centers thus risk losing kidney offers by listing too many marginal antigens to increase the calculated sensitization. Second, the antigen-specific information screens out some potential matches that would be considered on the basis of the PRA test but precluded by a positive crossmatch. Avoiding positive crossmatches reduces the cold ischemic time of donated kidneys and the costs of transplants by reducing the number of subsequent offers made to place the kidney. Third, by identifying specific antigens, the CPRA method permits more accurate assessments of African American and other minority sensitizations, generally increasing estimated sensitivity. Because the current and proposed kidney allocation systems put positive weight on sensitization, they have the potential to reduce racial disparity.

The Initial Kidney Allocation System

The Task Force on Organ Transplantation recognized that heavy reliance on HLA matching could potentially disadvantage minority patients: "It is important to safeguard against the risk of reducing access of certain segments of the population to renal transplantation by implementing mandated organ-sharing programs. In a system that shares organs on the basis of histocompatibility testing, patients are at a disadvantage whose HLA types either are not currently well defined or are different from the donor population" (1986, 92).

The task force also expressed concern that HLA-based matching of donated kidneys to patients on a national list would divert kidneys from local areas with a majority of black patients and decrease the incentive of transplant centers in those areas to seek donations. Overall, the task force recommended that "organ-sharing programs that are designed to improve the probability of success be implemented in the interests of the effective and efficient use of organs and justice, and the effect of mandated organ sharing be constantly assessed to identify and rectify imbalances that might reduce access of any group" (1986, 92).

J. Michael Dennis describes the goal set out by the task force as *procedural justice*—providing equal opportunity for receiving a transplant no matter where one lives (1992, 133). The mechanism for achieving this goal is to share some organs nationally and the others through rules that are the same across local jurisdictions. He contrasts this goal to several others with which it must compete. *Medical efficiency* seeks to maximize graft and patient survival and implies national sharing with HLA matching to the extent the latter is clinically relevant—as discussed in chapter 7, one might also interpret medical efficiency in more explicitly utilitarian terms such as maximizing the gain in life years from the available supply of organs. *Supply efficiency* seeks to maximize the number of donated organs and implies local distribution to maintain incentives for transplant centers to recover as many organs as possible. *Medical justice*, as specifically set out by Congress in the National Organ Transplant Act, seeks to give highly sensitized patients greater chances of receiving transplants and implies that extra weight be given to these patients. *Sociological justice*, not to be confused with social value as applied in the early allocation of dialysis, seeks to equalize access across demographic groups and implies greater weight in allocation for longer waiting times. He also notes the various conflicts that arise among these goals—the sorts of conflicts inherent in almost all areas of public policy (Stone 2002; Weimer and Vining 2005). Most relevant to racial disparity, he notes that both efficiency in supply and medical efficiency conflict with sociological justice for African Americans.

Consistent with the view of the task force that cadaveric organs be viewed as a national resource and allocated according to the goal of procedural fairness, as well as the goals of medical efficiency, supply efficiency, and medical justice, the OPTN established the Organ Procurement and Distribution Committee to develop standard national allocation rules in the context of the geographical hierarchy that gives priority to patients in the locale the kidneys were harvested. Patients were added to the local waiting list by their transplant center and then to the national list maintained by UNOS. To increase their chances of receiving locally allocated kidneys, some patients would list at centers in more than one locality, a practice that continues today. The general OPTN approach was to try to standardize the criteria for local allocation and limit national sharing of kidneys to those for which the recipient and donor shared the six HLA antigens at the A, B, and DR loci. Even with national sharing of kidneys with six HLA matches, a payback system in place for voluntary sharing required that the centers receiving the kidneys subsequently pay back the centers sending them with kidneys that would otherwise be transplanted locally. As noted, organ procurement organizations (OPOs) could apply for variances from the allocation rules and many did—fifteen kidney allocation variances, most reducing the weight placed on HLA matching, were in effect within the first year after the rules went into effect (Abt Associates 1990, 91). Consequently, considerable cross-locale variation emerged over time in the criteria actually used for local allocation.

The development of the standard kidney allocation rules revealed disagreement over the importance of HLA matching for graft success. Two transplant luminaries represented different views. Thomas Starzl, who pioneered many transplant techniques, first at the University of Colorado and then at the University of Pittsburgh, proposed an allocation system that placed only moderate weight on HLA matching. Paul Terasaki, who made important contributions to tissue typing at UCLA, proposed a system with much greater weight on HLA matching. At its October 1987 meeting, one of the first for UNOS as OPTN administrator, the Starzl allocation system, already in use by the University of Pittsburgh since 1985, was adopted. It gave as many as twelve points for six HLA matches, but also as many as ten points for sensitivity and ten for relative time on the waiting list (Starzl et al. 1987). In February 1989, however, the OPTN adopted an alternative system advocated by Terasaki. It made two changes relevant to racial disparity. On the one hand, it awarded points in local allocation not on the bases of HLA matches but rather on the absence of mismatches, which Terasaki believed to be the relevant factor for graft success. Because minorities tend to have disproportionately large numbers of blanks, this change marginally reduced racial disparity in allocation. On the other hand, the Terasaki system increased the potential for racial disparity by placing much greater weight on HLA matching relative to waiting time and sensitization. For example, where zero HLA mismatches gave ten points, time on waiting list provided at most one point.

In a critique written shortly after the move to the Terasaki system, Starzl, Shapiro, and Teperman expressed fear that "a small group of determined lobbyists" (the advocates of tissue typing) had created a presumption that typing counts, despite mixed evidence (1989, 3433). (Generally, single-center studies tended to find little or no graft survival benefit from HLA matching, whereas studies that pooled together larger samples did.) Starzl and his colleagues feared a number of undesirable social consequences, including reduced fairness in access because of less emphasis on waiting time, would result. In a particularly strong statement, they noted that "typing itself, while perpetuating the dreams and ambitions of a few hundred or a few thousand typers or transplant surgeons and physicians, will become an instrument of social injustice to the extent that the distribution patterns are distorted. The first question to be asked is if ethnic minorities, specifically blacks, will be placed at a disadvantage by the new emphasis on matching" (3433–34.) This question began to be answered very soon after Starzl and colleagues posed it.

Racial Disparity in Kidney Allocation

Empirical research exploring the implications of HLA matching for African Americans began to appear shortly after the adoption of the new kidney allocation rules (Greenstein et al. 1989; Lazda and Blaesing 1989). Data collected in regions with variances to the standardized allocation rules soon provided a basis for looking specifically at the role of HLA matching. For example, the Regional Organ Bank of Illinois operated under a variance that gave no points for the absence of HLA-A mismatches, fewer points for the absence of HLA-B and HLA-R mismatches, and more points for waiting time. Relative to the standardized allocation rules, the variance increased the kidneys going to blacks by 5 percentage points, raising the proportion of black transplant recipients to nearly their proportion on the waiting list (Lazda 1991).

Even as early as 1990, it appeared that a majority of transplant professionals were skeptical of the appropriateness of giving allocation points for less than six HLA matches. Abt Associates surveyed 218 UNOS members about their perceptions of HLA matching in an evaluation of the OPTN it conducted for the Health Resources and Services Administration (1990). The analysts found that 65 percent of respondents overall (57 percent for histocompatibility personnel and 67 percent for transplant center personnel) believed that the point system should not favor matches in which there are fewer than four matches. Only 19 percent, however, believed that "HLA matching should not be a criterion for kidney sharing" (80).

During 1990 the HHS Office of Inspector General conducted a study of organ allocation. It found that on average blacks waited almost twice as long for a kidney transplant as whites, even controlling for blood type, age, and location (Office of Inspector General 1991). The report recommended that OPOs be required to create unified lists of patients awaiting transplantation and that, "subject to established medical criteria," organs be distributed on a first-come, first-served basis (iii). In other words, the report supported the use of waiting time as the primary basis for kidney allocation.

A comprehensive and ultimately influential case against heavy reliance on HLA matching was made by two law professors, Ian Ayres and Laura Dooley, and a transplant surgeon, Robert Gaston, in 1993. In an article in the *Vanderbilt Law Review*, they drew together available medical evidence to argue against the standardized point system, especially the weight given to HLA matching, because of its disparate impact on African Americans (Ayers et al. 1993; see also Gaston et al. 1993). After arguing that the benefits of HLA matching were uncertain and most likely declining, they noted that the OPTN had already shown a willingness to sacrifice medical efficiency for medical justice in the priority points awarded to highly sensitized patients, which increases the rate of second transplants that are generally less successful, and the limitation of O-type kidneys to O-type patients, even though it would be medically appropriate to allocate them to patients with other blood types. They proposed modifying the allocation rules to eliminate points for two or more HLA mismatches, doubling the points awarded for waiting time, and providing additional points for those with rare antigens. In the following year, the OPTN adopted several of the proposals Ayers and his colleagues had made (1993).

Incremental Responses

In the years following the introduction of the initial standardized kidney allocation rules, the OPTN considered a number of changes to reduce racial disparity. Two of these changes, adopted in 1994 and 2002, reduced the importance of HLA matching. Two other changes were adopted as local options: the allocation of A_2 blood type kidneys to B blood type patients and the calculation of waiting time based on initiation of dialysis rather than placement on the waiting list. Yet another series of changes shifted priority for mandatorily shared kidneys. These incremental changes mirrored the gradual evolution of liver allocation rules before the model for end-stage liver disease (MELD) was adopted, as discussed in chapter 5.

1994 HLA Changes

The OPTN began a general review of allocation policies with the creation of the Ad Hoc Committee on Organ Allocation in 1993. The committee circulated a document for public comment at the end of 1993 and held public forums on it in January and February of 1994. It revised the document and circulated it for comment among the standing OPTN committees. At the June board of directors meeting, the *UNOS Statement of Principles and Objectives of Equitable Organ Allocation* was adopted (UNOS 1994b). It calls for a balancing among supply efficiency, medical efficiency, medical justice, and respect for the autonomy of persons. One of the ten objectives set out to further these principles is to minimize disparities in waiting time among patients with similar medical or demographic characteristics.

At the same meeting, the board of directors split the Organ Procurement and Distribution Committee into the Kidney/Pancreas Committee, the Thoracic Committee, and the Liver/Intestinal Organ Committee. The previous arrangement had reflected the dominance of kidney allocation at the time the OPTN was created. With the growing importance of the transplantation of livers, pancreases, and intestines, the Organ Procurement and Distribution Committee had created subcommittees to focus on issues specific to these organs. The 1994 changes reorganized these subcommittees and the parent committee into three parallel committees that have since evolved into the primary arenas for considering the substance of allocation rules.

The question of the importance of HLA matching for graft success was addressed by the Histocompatibility Committee during 1994. The committee worked with UNOS staff to analyze data from the almost thirty thousand kidney transplants recorded in the Scientific Registry of Transplant Recipients from its initiation in October 1987 through 1991. Multivariate models of patient and graft survival were estimated to control statistically for factors such as donor and recipient age, cold ischemic time, PRA score, and comorbidities. The models provided two very important results (UNOS 1994a, 18). First, relative to four or more mismatches, zero mismatches at the HLA-A and HLA-B loci did not make a statistically significant contribution to graft success. Second, zero HLA mismatches made the same contribution to graft success as six HLA matches. It thus appeared that the elimination of points for zero mismatches at the HLA-A and HLA-B loci and the switch to zero HLA mismatches for mandatory sharing, both of which had potential to reduce the disadvantage in access of African Americans, could be done without reducing medical efficiency.

The Histocompatibility Committee recommended to the board of directors that the standardized allocation rules be modified to reflect these findings. At its June meeting, the board of directors decided to send out the proposed changes for public comment. At its November meeting the board approved the recommendations, which were implemented in March 1995. Subsequently, the board approved doubling the points given for each year on the waiting list and increasing the points award for pediatric status; these latter changes were effective July 1995. Table 6–2 summarizes these changes. The 1994 column shows the allocation system in place at the end of that year and the 1995–2002 column shows the revised allocation system.

A_2 and A_2B Allocation

As shown in table 6–1, African American ESRD patients awaiting transplants have blood type B at almost twice the rate as the donor population. Strict allocation within the ABO blood boundaries reduces the chances that African American patients with blood type B receive cadaveric kidneys. Clinical experiments done before the operation of the OPTN showed that the ABO blood barrier was not absolute. Most significantly, beginning in 1986, the Midwest Organ Bank started clinical trials in which A_2 and A_2B kidneys were transplanted into B and O patients. In 1991, the Midwest Organ Bank received a variance from the OPTN that allowed it to preferentially allocate A_2 kidneys first to B and then to O patients. In 1994 it obtained a modified variance allowing it to give priority to sensitized A_1 and A_1B patients before B and O patients. A study of the fifty cross-barrier transplants done between 1986 and 1996 found no clinical difference in outcomes for B and O patients meeting certain immunological conditions (Nelson et al. 1998). In June 2000 the Texas Organ Sharing Alliance also received a variance to allocate A_2 and A_2B kidneys to B and O patients.

The Minority Affairs Committee reviewed the published research and concluded that a larger study was needed to assess more fully the impacts of allocating A_2 and A_2B kidneys to B and O patients on graft success and access to transplantation for A and B patients. At its March 2000 meeting, the committee chair appointed a subcommittee to develop a proposal for a voluntary variance that would allow OPOs to participate in a coordinated study. The proposal was subsequently sent to the board of directors, which sent it out for comment in March 2001 and approved it in June 2001.

The Minority Affairs Committee continues to monitor the data generated under the national voluntary variance. By the end of 2006, ten OPOs were participating in the variance and data on forty-three transplants involving A_2 and A_2B kidneys to B patients had been collected. Three-quarters of these transplant recipients were minorities, although almost as many were Asian Americans as African Americans (twelve versus fourteen). At the request of the committee, UNOS staff analyzed the accumulated data and confirmed the findings of the earlier studies that graft and patient survival rates for these types of transplants were comparable to those involving B kidneys to B patients (Cherikh and Cheng 2007). These accumulating findings are providing a strong basis for eventually making the variance mandatory.

Table 6–2   Kidney Allocation Rules

Category	1994	1995–2002	2003
"Mandatory share"[a]	6 HLA matches	0 HLA mismatches	0 HLA mismatches
Allocation points			
0 A, B or DR mismatches	10	—	—
0 B or DR mismatches	7	7	—
0 A or B mismatches	6	—	—
1 B or DR mismatch	3	5	—
2 B or DR mismatches	2	2	—
3 B or DR mismatches	1	—	—
0 DR mismatches	—	—	2
1 DR mismatches	—	—	1
Sensitization (PRA>0.79)[b]	4	4	4
Longest waiting time[c]	1	1	1
Each full year waiting	0.5	1	1
Patient younger than eleven[d]	3	4	4
Patient age 11 to 18[d]	2	3	3
Patient prior live donor	—	4[e]	4

Source: Author's compilation.

[a] Offered first locally, then regionally, then nationally; allocation based on points when multiple matches within geographic level; requires destination OPO to pay back origin OPO with a kidney in the future.
[b] Assumes negative cross-match between donor and potential recipient.
[c] Full point awarded to patient with donor blood type who has longest waiting time; fractions of points awarded to those waiting shorter times; for example, if ten patients were waiting for a type-O kidney, then the patient waiting the third longest would receive 0.8 points.
[d] Pediatric patients receive priority for kidneys from donors younger than thirty-five over all others except sensitized patients.
[e] Introduced in 1996.

2002 HLA Changes

Concern about the implications of favoring partial HLA matches on racial disparity in access to kidney transplantation remained even after the changes adopted in 1994. Evaluations of those changes generally concluded that only the change in mandatory national sharing from six HLA matches to zero HLA mismatches contributed to an increase in transplants for African Americans (Zachary et al. 1997; Hata et al. 1998; Laffell and Zachary 1999). However, an evaluation of a variance used in UNOS Region 1 (New England) that eliminated points for other-than-zero mismatches at the HLA-B and HLA-DR loci suggested that further reductions in the weight placed on HLA matching would increase minority access to transplants. Critics continued to question the desirability of assigning any points based on more than zero HLA mismatches (Young and Gaston 2000).

Throughout the late 1990s the board of directors addressed concerns about racial disparity in kidney transplantation. In addition to the variance allowing blood type B patients to receive A_2 and A_2B kidneys, the board also authorized a pilot study of the effect of basing allocation on cross-reactive antigen groups (CREGs), families of related antigens, rather than specific HLA antigens. For example, under CREG matching, antigens numbered 15 and 16 would be considered equivalent to the antigen numbered 2 at the HLA-DR locus (OPTN 2007, appendix 3A). Basing matching on CREGs potentially reduces the disadvantage minorities with rare antigens face because these rare antigens are considered to be members of families that contain more common antigens (McKenna and Takemoto 2000). Finding a match within a CREG is thus more likely than finding one among the individual antigens.

The board of directors also recognized the value of increasing its analytical capacity for assessing rule changes. As discussed in chapter 5, the UNOS liver allocation model played an important role in assessing the consequences of wider geographic sharing of livers. The kidney transplant community expressed a desire to have a similar simulation tool available. In response, the board appointed the Kidney Allocation Modeling Oversight Committee to guide the development of what became the UNOS Kidney Allocation Model (UKAM[SM]) by UNOS staff and Symex Systems, a consulting firm (Taranto et al. 2000). The model allows simulations of alternative rules based on either patients actually added to the waiting list and actual donors during an historical period, beginning in 1996 and extending forward, or data generated according to expectations about the future composition of patients and donors. In 2000, after substantial validation, the Kidney Allocation Oversight Committee voted to begin using the model to assess alternative allocation rules.

The interest of both the Minority Affairs Committee and the Kidney and Pancreas Transplantation Committee (KPTC) in the HLA issue led to the formation of a joint subcommittee, which also included the chair of the Histocompatibility Committee, to develop possible revisions to the kidney allocation rules. The subcommittee met during the first half of 2001. It made extensive use of the UKAM[SM] to consider a wide range of possible rule changes. The analyses suggested that both reducing the emphasis on HLA matching and increasing the geographic extent of sharing areas would increase somewhat the number of African American patients receiving transplants. It would also increase the percentages of repeat, pediatric, and highly sensitized patients receiving transplants. These changes would have only small negative effects on graft success.

Although expanding the geographic extent of sharing appeared to offer as large an increase as reduced emphasis on HLA matching, the subcommittee rejected the former because of what its members perceived as limitations of the UKAM^{SM} with respect to its assumptions about crossmatching. Specifically, it expected that transplant centers would not be willing to accept a kidney for a highly sensitized patient without a preliminary negative crossmatch. However, the infrastructure for doing the preliminary crossmatching currently exists only at the local level, and the methods used vary considerably from one locale to another, so that these crossmatches would not actually be available. Consequently, the committee viewed the model results as overly optimistic. This episode clearly illustrates how tacit knowledge based on direct experience in the transplant system tempers evidence-based quantitative analysis in OPTN deliberations.

The subcommittee also rejected wider geographic sharing because it anticipated that this more radical change would encounter substantial resistance, based at least in part on concerns about the implications for procurement efforts. Rather, it opted for an incremental strategy and the continued collecting of evidence to set the stage for possible additional changes in the future.

In July 2001 the subcommittee voted 5 to 1 in favor of proposing the elimination of HLA-related points in allocation. That is, other than the mandatory sharing of zero HLA mismatched kidneys, HLA matching would no longer play a role in allocation. As shown in the third column of table 6–2, zero mismatches at the HLA-B and HLA-DR loci then received seven points. Given that this is equivalent in terms of priority to a patient being on the waiting list for seven years, the proposed change was substantial. The subcommittee explicitly recognized the value trade-off inherent in the proposal: "As with the kidney allocation system overall, a decision to retain or modify HLA match points requires a balance among factors of medical utility and justice. The joint subcommittee determined that in this case the balance favors a change that can remove a factor in the system resulting in disparate benefit among patient populations with mitigated harm as a result of advances in science and medicine" (UNOS 2001, 33). The KPTC voted 15 to 2 to support distribution of the proposal for public comment.

The public comment was on balance negative. Of the 194 responses received, 27 percent supported the proposal, 60 percent opposed it, and 12 percent expressed no opinion (UNOS 2002a, 6). Responses from other OPTN committees were mixed, but on the whole negative, and seven of the eleven UNOS regions voted against it. Three major criticisms of the proposal were voiced. First, as acknowledged by the subcommittee, the proposal would cause a small decrease in graft survival. Some feared that this small effect would cumulate into a substantial effect over time. Second, because more patients would receive kidneys with more mismatches, sensitization would become even more severe for those needing a second transplant. Third, the proposal would not adequately reduce the disparities it is intended to address. In November 2001, the KPTC referred the proposal back to the subcommittee for further consideration.

In March of 2002, the American Society of Transplantation, the American Society of Transplant Surgeons, the Association of Organ Procurement Organizations, the Scientific Registry of Transplant Recipients (SRTR), and UNOS sponsored the National Conference on the Wait List for Kidney Transplantation. Analysts from the SRTR presented data suggesting that for kidney transplants since 1995, mismatches at the HLA-B locus appeared to have a small effect on graft failure—two mismatches increased the failure risk by only 7 percent relative to zero mismatches and one mismatch appeared to have the same risk as zero mismatches (Gaston et al. 2003). These data led to a conference proposal to eliminate points for HLA-B mismatches but to keep points for HLA-DR mismatches.

The subcommittee worked with SRTR staff to produce a number of analyses to assess this modification of its original proposal. A multivariate analysis of more than thirty-two thousand kidney recipients showed that, though increasing mismatches at any of the three HLA loci increased the risk of graft failure, only mismatches at the HLA-DR locus had statistically significant effects. Waiting list analysis indicated that eliminating points for HLA-B mismatches would result in increases in transplants for black, Asian, and Hispanic patients of 8 percent, 7 percent, and 5 percent, respectively; transplants to white patients would decrease by 6 percent (UNOS 2002b, 8). These percentage gains for minorities were only slightly smaller than those expected under the original proposal. Consequently, much of the expected benefit could be gained and reductions in graft success avoided by only eliminating HLA-B points.

Other analyses considered the risk of increased sensitization that might result from first transplants with less well-matched kidneys. The general findings were that mismatch at first transplant probably was not having as large an effect on sensitization as widely feared. Any mismatch appeared to increase the risk of sensitization relative to zero mismatches at all three HLA loci, but there appeared to be no systematic differentiation among the number of mismatches at the HLA-B and HLA-DR loci. Some members of the subcommittee speculated that the lack of a relationship might result from random distribution of HLA-A matches after they were removed from the allocation system. Overall, the subcommittee concluded that risks of increased sensitization should not be a major concern. Finally, the subcommittee analyzed data from two OPOs and a region that had variances to operate alternative allocation systems that de-emphasized HLA matching relative to the standard allocation rules. Data from these locales suggested that increases in minority access did actually result and that there appeared to be no increase in graft failure.

The question remained about how many points to assign to HLA-DR mismatches. The KPTC was concerned about leaving too much weight on mismatches. As patients spend on average about three years on the waiting list before a transplant, thereby accumulating about three points, the subcommittee decided to propose that zero mismatches accrue two points and one mismatch accrues one point. The vote on this point allocation was 9 to 0 with 3 abstentions. Both the Minority Affairs Committee and the KPTC subsequently voted unanimously to seek public comment on the revised proposal. Public comment was solicited in August 2002.

One of the major public criticisms of the proposal was that the new point allocation was arbitrary. As a compromise to move the change forward, the KPTC submitted a revised proposal to the board of directors that retained the higher point allocations that would be consistent with the existing allocation system: seven points for zero HLA-DR mismatches and five points for one HLA-DR mismatch. However, new data presented at the November 2002 meeting of the board of directors suggested that these allocations would actually reduce transplantation access for African Americans. In response the proposal was amended to return to the smaller allocations. That is, two points for zero HLA-DR mismatches and one for one HLA-DR mismatch (see table 6–2, column 3). The board approved the amended proposal on an interim basis and called for an expeditious re-evaluation of the point allocations. By May 2003 both the KPTC and the Minority Affairs Committee completed favorable reviews of the change based on SRTR reports and voted to support the proposal as adopted by the board.

Waiting Time Definition

Patients become eligible for the kidney transplantation waiting list when either their kidney function declines below a minimum threshold (a creatinine clearance level of less than or equal to twenty milliliters per minute) or they begin dialysis. About 80 percent of patients on the waiting list are listed sometime after they have begun dialysis. The remaining patients are listed preemptively, that is, before they have begun dialysis. Preemptive listing creates an opportunity for receiving a transplant before dialysis is initiated, which increases the chances of graft success. Preemptive listing and transplantation are especially valuable for pediatric patients because dialysis interferes with growth and development.

Disparities in access to kidney transplantation begin in the listing process. Black patients on dialysis are referred for evaluation, evaluated, and placed on the kidney transplant waiting list at lower rates than white patients (Epstein et al. 2003). Blacks who are listed tend to be listed after a longer time on dialysis (Furth et al. 2000; Danovitch, Cohen, and Smits 2002). Controlling for type of insurance and a number of patient characteristics, blacks are listed on average 233 days later and their odds of preemptive listing are less than half those of white patients (Keith et al. 2008). Although there are some racial differences in preferences for, and expectations about, kidney transplantation, these differences explain only a small fraction of the disparities in access to transplantation (Ayanian et al. 1999). Recognizing these disparities, the National Conference on the Wait List for Kidney Transplantation recommended that waiting time for kidney allocation be calculated based on when the patient begins dialysis rather than on when the patient is added to the waiting list (Gaston et al. 2003, 779). The KPTC began consideration of this recommendation at its May 2002 meeting, referring the issue to the joint subcommittee to consider along with HLA-related issues. The subcommittee recommended that a proposal to make the change be sent out for public comments. Signaling the heated controversy that would arise over this issue, the motion to recommend the proposal to the board of directors passed by an unusually close vote of 8 to 6.

Public comments on the proposal were requested in August 2002. Those opposing the proposal raised a number of objections. Some critics pointed out that the proposal deals with only one aspect of the listing disparity, but ignores the perhaps more serious problems of appropriate transplant candidates never being listed or listed after long periods of dialysis that reduce their chances of successful grafts. Other critics noted inconsistencies of the proposal with other components of the kidney allocation system. Most important, the proposal seemed at odds with the rules then in place regarding the accrual of waiting time for patients listed as inactive, say because they had a temporary medical condition that made them ineligible for a transplant. These patients received a maximum of thirty days toward waiting time during their inactive period. In contrast, under the proposal someone could receive a credit of several years for the period in which they were ineligible for a transplant because they had not been evaluated and placed on the waiting list. (This potential inconsistency was subsequently removed in June 2003 when the board of directors changed the rules to allow for the continued accrual of waiting time no matter how long the patient was listed as inactive; at the same meeting the board approved the reinstatement of waiting time for those whose grafts fail within three months.)

The KPTC was unable to reach agreement on moving the proposal forward when it met to respond to the public comments in October 2002. Rather, it decided to request that SRTR analysts provide more information on the distribution of impacts. The analysis indicated that across all patients, the average accrued waiting time would increase by 1.3 years. Black patients would see an increase on average of 1.7 years, whites one of 1.2 years, and Hispanics of 1.6 years. (Subsequent analysis determined that most of the gain for Hispanics was for white Hispanics.) If pediatric patients were included (they were inadvertently excluded from the original proposal), then they would gain on average only about 0.8 years, primarily because the point allocation under existing rules was designed to increase the chances that they would receive transplants before they began dialysis. Diabetics, who generally do less well on dialysis and are often listed before beginning dialysis, would gain on average 1.1 years.

After modifying the proposal to include pediatric patients and making it clear that the proposal would still allow the accumulation of waiting time from the point of preemptive listing, the committee voted 10 to 4 to resubmit the proposal for public comment. However, at their meetings in January 2003, the Minority Affairs Committee raised concerns about a possible disadvantage for diabetic patients and the Pediatric Transplantation Committee raised concerns about a possible disadvantage for pediatric patients. In response, the KPTC decided to ask the SRTR for an updated analysis to help assess the concerns that were raised. Although the pediatric concerns were not fully allayed—some adults would gain four or more points so that they would potentially move ahead of some pediatric patients—the committee decided at its July 2002 meeting that this problem should be addressed by increasing the points awarded to pediatric patients rather than holding up the proposal. Similarly, the committee thought it best to deal with any disadvantages for diabetics in a separate proposal. It voted 20 to 1 with 1 abstention to reaffirm its earlier decision to send the proposal out again for public comment.

The call for public comments in August 2003 again elicited mixed and heated responses including some from patients on the waiting list who feared the change would move others ahead of them in terms of accumulated waiting time points—Alan Leichtman, who was chair of the KPTC during this period, recounted receiving death threats related to the proposal at the March 12, 2008, meeting of the Kidney Transplantation Committee attended by the author. The KPTC responded to the continued opposition to the proposal by changing it from a modification of the standardized allocation rules to a committee-sponsored alternative allocation system like that used for A_2 and A_2B allocation. At its November 2003 meeting the board of directors initially accepted the proposal but later in the meeting rescinded it in favor of a voluntary pilot study. That study began in 2006 with two participating OPOs.

Priority for Mandatory Shares

About 14 percent of transplants involve mandatory sharing of zero HLA mismatched kidneys. The 1994 change from six HLA matches to zero HLA mismatches increased the access of African Americans to mandatory shares. A number of subsequent marginal changes to mandatory share allocations have been adopted to increase access for minority, sensitized, and pediatric patients.

In June 2001 the board of directors eliminated the priority given to positive matches among those with zero mismatches. Instead, allocation of mandatorily shared kidneys at each geographic level was to depend on sensitization and then waiting time, a change intended to further increase minority access to mandatory shares. In November 2002 the board extended priority for adult sensitized patients to include those with 21 to 79 percent PRA. At the following meeting in June 2003, the board clarified that highly sensitized pediatric patients (PRAs greater than 79 percent) received priority after highly sensitized adult patients but before moderately sensitized adult patients.

Other changes related to mandatory sharing involve the complications that arise from combined pancreas and kidney transplants, expanded-criteria-donor kidneys, and payback policies. It is enough to be aware that they complicate the allocation system and create the potential for rule changes to have indirect consequences. They are worth noting for two reasons. First, although many readers who, like the author, are not part of the transplantation enterprise probably find the discussion of incremental changes already discussed as quite complex, reality is even more complicated—sitting in on a committee meeting or reading a committee transcript makes this very evident. Committees like the KPTC can function so well in the face of great complexity only because they consist primarily of people who are involved professionally in transplantation on a day-to-day basis and who become involved in the work of the committee for several years at a time. Second, the committees produce continuous incremental change reflecting experience with previous changes as well as scientific and clinical knowledge. This incremental change, though, has substantially increased the complexity of the kidney allocation system, making its operation less transparent to patients.

Conclusion

Change is difficult whenever the status quo has a self-identified constituency. Patients who expect to receive a kidney soon under the current allocation rules are a strong constituency for keeping those rules. It is not surprising that changing the kidney allocation rules required considerable effort and often involved substantial delay during which evidence could be marshaled to make cases strong enough to overcome the bias for maintaining the status quo. Unfortunately, these incremental changes were from a starting point that produced considerable racial disparity in access to kidney transplantation. Despite the progress made through the various incremental changes, it would be hard to argue that, even in view of the competing values, the remaining racial disparity should be ignored. Nonetheless, the OPTN governance arrangements have kept the issue prominent. The

KPTC identified specific alternatives that could potentially address the disparity. It assessed the consequences of these alternatives with analyses involving intensive use of data and sophisticated models as well as tacit knowledge from participants in the transplant system. It consulted both internally and externally with interested parties and advanced the most promising alternatives through the formal decision-making process. Whereas someone concerned about social justice outcomes would likely be disappointed with the progress so far, someone familiar with regulatory and other governmental decision-making processes as they actually operate would likely find solace that change in the desirable direction occurred and is likely to continue to occur.

7

The Kidney Allocation Review
Can the OPTN Make Nonincremental Change?

The modifications made to liver allocation rules during the Final Rule controversy and to kidney allocation rules in response to concerns about racial disparity show the capacity of the OPTN for using statistical evidence, working with the SRTR to conduct sophisticated policy simulations, confronting value conflicts, and assessing the tacit knowledge of transplant professionals to support and make incremental change. In the case of liver allocation, the cumulative effects of the incremental changes eventually resulted in a substantially different allocation system. In the case of kidney allocation, a large number of small changes were made within the framework of the original system. Although continuous incremental change in socially valued directions is certainly a desirable feature of any form of medical governance, the capacity to make more fundamental change, either to respond to new challenges or to make faster progress toward recognized goals, is also desirable. What is the capacity of the OPTN for making nonincremental change? The recently implemented lung allocation policy shows that such change is possible. However, an assessment of the more challenging efforts of the OPTN begun in 2004 to conduct a comprehensive review and possible redesign of the kidney allocation system provides a more substantial basis for answering this question.

An appropriate starting point in considering nonincremental change is its definition in the context of organ allocation. I consider a nonincremental change to an organ allocation system to be one that substantially alters both its underlying values and the methods for pursuing them. The model for end-stage liver disease and pediatric end-stage liver disease (MELD/PELD) revisions in the liver allocation system were major changes in methods for determining medical urgency, but not a departure from medical urgency as the primary underlying value. The modifications to the kidney allocation system discussed in chapter 6 substantially changed neither the methods nor the underlying values, but rather shifted somewhat the relative weight placed on promoting the underlying values of medical efficiency and equity of access.

What motivated the efforts for achieving nonincremental change in kidney allocation? A comprehensive review of the kidney allocation system is consistent with the responsibility given to the OPTN in the Final Rule to review and revise allocation policies periodically to seek to achieve the best use of donated organs, including avoiding waste and futile transplants, and to promote patient access. However, one might reasonably argue

117

that the OPTN routinely reviews and revises kidney allocation rules. Several other considerations were probably more important in launching the effort. The underlying values, medical efficacy narrowly defined in terms of graft success based on antigen matching, and equity of access, as reflected in the weight placed on waiting time, did not necessarily yield the best use of kidneys if one considers such values as medical benefit as potentially relevant. As should be clear from the discussion in chapter 6, the various incremental changes to the kidney allocation system make it decidedly complex: payback rules linked to mandatory sharing, dual systems of rules for standard and extended criteria kidneys, a variance for A_2 and A_2B allocation, to name just a few of the factors complicating the stylized point system. In addition to ongoing concerns about racial disparity in access, there were growing concerns about the waste resulting from rejection of offered payback and extended criteria kidneys. Finally, the revisions of the liver, and especially the lung, allocation rules provided precedents for substantial change.

After a brief review of the redesign of the lung allocation system, this chapter considers the development of a proposal for a nonincremental change in kidney allocation. It focuses on the operation of the committee system in gathering and assessing information during the development process and thus offers yet another look at the process of decision making within the OPTN.

The Precedent: Redesign of the Lung Allocation System

In 1990 the OPTN first addressed the allocation of isolated lungs, those not transplanted along with their donor's heart. Priority within a geographic zone was determined by time on the waiting list for patients whose blood type matched the donated lungs. Patients at transplant centers served by the OPO that recovered the lungs received the highest geographic priority. Following the convention used for heart allocation, priority after local allocation was according to successive concentric zones with radii in five-hundred-nautical-mile increments. The only major change to this allocation system before 2005 was the addition of ninety days of waiting time credit for patients with idiopathic pulmonary fibrosis, a condition that contributed to increased mortality while on the waiting list.

In 1998, in anticipation of the requirements for periodic review to be imposed by the Final Rule, the Thoracic Organ Transplantation Committee (TOTC) agreed to reconsider the use of waiting time as the primary determinant of priority. The efforts that followed have been documented by the directly involved committee members and UNOS and SRTR staff (Egan et al. 2006). The following account of the process that led to the new allocation system implemented in 2005 is based primarily on this report (but see also OPTN 2005, chapter 9), which is an unusually rich recounting of organizational processes for an article published in a medical journal. Indeed, were these sorts of accounts more common, writing this book would have been much easier and perhaps less necessary.

In 1999 the TOTC formed a subcommittee to consider allocation systems based on urgency status rather than waiting time. The subcommittee, which eventually became the Lung Allocation Subcommittee, set out three goals for any new allocation system: "(1) reduction of mortality on the lung waiting list; (2) prioritization of candidates based on urgency while avoiding futile transplants; and (3) 'de-emphasizing the role of waiting time and geography in lung allocation within the limits of ischemic time'" (Egan et al. 2006, 1214). Working with SRTR staff, the subcommittee built models of time on waiting list and post-transplant survival as a basis for an allocation algorithm. It chose to base the models on objective clinical data that could not be easily manipulated by transplant centers to give their patients higher priorities. The subcommittee presented its initial proposal at the Conference on Lung Allocation Policy sponsored by the OPTN in March 2003. Although the proposal received general support from the conference participants, it also elicited a number of suggestions for revisions that the subcommittee incorporated into a proposal sent out for public comment in August 2003.

That proposal did not receive a warm reception from the broader transplant community, which raised a number of concerns (OPTN/SRTR 2005, chapter 9). First, although the committee envisioned that the survival scores would be routinely updated with data from new cohorts, this was not made clear enough to avoid complaints that the analysis relied on data that were too old. Second, within diagnostic groups some risk factors well established in the literature did not prove statistically or clinically significant: patients on the waiting list were usually already quite ill and thus some of the factors that were very relevant in determining the risk among all patients in the diagnostic group washed out of the analysis. Nonetheless, the failure of these risk factors to be statistically important made some transplant surgeons skeptical of the models. Third, some patient advocacy groups raised concerns that the modeling by diagnostic group might discriminate against their patients. Finally, members of the pediatric lung transplant community expressed concerns that the original proposal did not adequately take account of the special needs of the pediatric population.

The subcommittee and the TOTC revised and clarified the proposal in response to these concerns. Table 7–1 displays the allocation system that resulted. The key innovation, which qualifies it as a nonincremental change, is the weight placed on the transplant benefit, which is the difference between the predicted average number of days of life during the first year following a transplant minus the predicted average number of days of life during the next year on the waiting list. This is a utilitarian approach similar to the sort of net benefit calculation that would seem natural to economists but was not reflected in any of the organ allocation systems then in use. Transplant benefit was not the only factor included, however. Out of concern that basing allocation only on transplant net benefit would place too little weight on urgency, the proposal places equal weight on transplant benefit and waiting list urgency. Mathematically, this choice results in the raw allocation score being equivalent to the posttransplant survival measure minus twice the waiting list urgency measure—subtracted first to yield the net transplant benefit and second to give it equal weight to the net transplant benefit. This combined measure, the raw lung allocation score, theoretically ranges from 365 days (someone predicted to live a full year with a transplant and to die immediately without one) to −730 days (someone predicted to die immediately with a transplant but to live a full year on the waiting list). A linear normalization converts the raw lung allocation score to the normalized lung allocation score (LAS), which is the basis for allocation of lungs to patients twelve years old and older.

The OPTN board of directors unanimously approved the proposal in June 2004. The TOTC created a new subcommittee to guide implementation and authorized it to resolve

Table 7–1   2005 Lung Allocation System

Normalized lung allocation score (LAS)
LAS = (100) [(TB – WLUM) + 2 (365)]/[(3)(365)]
WLUM: waiting list urgency measure, the expected number of days lived without a transplant during an additional year on the waiting list calculated as the area under the appropriate one-year survival curve. Survival curves are estimated using multivariate hazard models for each of four major diagnostic groups (chronic obstructive pulmonary disease cystic fibrosis, primary pulmonary hypertension, and idiopathic pulmonary fibrosis). Survival curves for the 20 percent of cases with other diagnoses are estimated by pooling them with the most statistically similar of the four major diagnosis groups. The models are re-estimated every six months as new cohorts of data become available.
PTSM: posttransplant survival measure, the expected number of days lived during the first-year following transplantation calculated as the area under the appropriate one-year survival curve. As with WLUM, the PTSM is based on multivariate hazard models by diagnostic group. These models generally have fewer explanatory variables than the WLUM models. The models are also re-estimated every six months.
TB: transplant benefit, the difference between the posttransplant survival measure (PTSM) and the waiting list urgency measure (WLSM). TB is an estimate of the marginal gain from the patient receiving a transplant.
Other features
Pediatric allocation: patients younger than twelve receive priority by waiting time for lungs from donors younger than twelve. Lungs from donors age twelve to seventeen are allocated first to patients age twelve to seventeen by LAS, then to patients under twelve by waiting time, and finally to adult patients by LAS. The small number of patients younger than twelve prevented them from being confidently included in the WLUM and PTSM models. Matching donors and patients by age facilitates consideration of lungs of appropriate size.
Blood type: allocation is within the standard ABO blood groups.
Patient data: except for right heart catheterization data, patient data must be updated every six months. (Right heart catheterization is updated only at the discretion of the transplant center because it involves patient risk.)
Normalization: the various numbers in the LAS formula convert the raw scale, TB – WLUM or PTSM – 2WLUM, which theoretically ranges from –730 to 365, to a normalized score of between 0 and 100.

Source: Author's compilation based on Egan et al. 2006; OPTN/SRTR 2005, chapter 9.

any remaining issues that arose. For example, the subcommittee defined default values for any missing or out-of-date data needed to implement the LAS so that failure to report these data would not benefit patients. The TOTC also worked with the board to develop guidelines for a national Lung Review Board to consider requests from transplant centers for increasing the priority for patients with exceptional circumstances, say by using estimated rather than default values when data are missing.

The new system was implemented in May 2005. As with all the OPTN allocation systems, incremental modifications continue to be considered and adopted. Also, some criticisms of the LAS have been voiced. For example, because lung transplants can improve quality of life even when they do not contribute to longevity, some argue that LAS should incorporate a quality of life adjustment (Egan and Kotloff 2005, 413). Nonetheless, the approach embodied in the LAS has been greeted with general approval. It shows the possibility of nonincremental change by the OPTN. It also set precedents for several of the elements that emerged in the proposal for a nonincremental change of the kidney allocation system.

Efforts toward Fundamental Change: Kidney Allocation Based on Net Benefit

Between 2005 and 2008, the OPTN developed a nonincremental proposal that introduced maximizing net benefit, as measured by the gain in life years from transplant, as a substantial factor in kidney allocation. The following account views the development of the proposal from three perspectives. First, an overview of the process of developing the proposal notes the major activities and events during the four years over which the proposal was developed. Second, a breakdown of the major components of the proposal, and what influenced their design, reveals its substance. Third, a sketch of the pattern of organizational interaction conveys the extensive collaboration involved in developing a well-specified proposal.

Process Overview

Although the origins of policy proposals are usually difficult to pin down, it would not be unreasonable to point to a discussion of the net benefit concept at the July 2003 meeting of the Kidney and Pancreas Transplantation Committee as the analytical starting point for the new kidney allocation system. (The Kidney and Pancreas Transplantation Committee was split into the Kidney Transplantation Committee and the Pancreas Transplantation Committee in 2006. The acronym KTC is used in this chapter to refer first to the Kidney and Pancreas Transplantation Committee and then to the Kidney Transplantation Committee.) Robert Wolfe, an SRTR analyst, presented the idea of basing kidney allocation on the principle of maximizing net benefits by allocating each available kidney to the patient for whom it would yield the largest net benefit. He noted that one implementation of net benefit could be based on estimates of the difference in life years with and without a transplant for each patient, giving priority to the patient with the largest net gain. Another implementation could be based on estimates of survival times without a transplant, giving priority to the patient with the shortest survival time, as is effectively done in liver allocation.

The KTC continued discussion of the net benefit principle at its next meeting the following October. A variety of views were expressed. Some members were concerned that a net benefit principle would place too much weight on utility at the expense of medical justice. Others raised concern about the difficulty of reducing net benefit to a specific number. These discussions showed a lack of consensus about the need for a fundamental change in the approach to kidney allocation. Nonetheless, in a vote of 20 to 2, the committee endorsed the proposal that future modeling efforts consider net benefits.

The capacity for modeling was being enhanced through the development of the Kidney-Pancreas Simulated Allocation Model (KPSAM). At the request of the Health Resources and Services Administration, the SRTR created a family of flexible simulation models for assessing liver, heart, lung, kidney, and pancreas allocation polices (Thompson et al. 2004). The models simulate the arrival of both organs and patients with specific sets of characteristics to the transplantation system. Statistical relationships estimated using historical data provide the basis for translating these characteristics into changes in status, such as removal from the waiting list because of death. Policy experiments involve comparing the simulation outcomes under alternative allocation rules. These policy experiments became the analytical workhorses during the development of the net benefit proposal.

In November 2003 the board of directors adopted a resolution requiring all organ committees to assess proposals to the board in terms of compliance with the provisions of the Final Rule, including performance goals and performance measures. The KTC began discussion of its response to the resolution at its January 2004 meeting. Members started by discussing whether the call in the Final Rule for emphasis on medical urgency applied to end-stage renal disease (ESRD), which, unlike the diseases affecting other organs, had an alternative life-preserving treatment, namely dialysis. The call in the Final Rule for separate allocation systems for different organs was interpreted as allowing a flexible interpretation of medical urgency. The discussion continued at the May meeting. Some members argued that the goal should be a fair system that is as simple and open as possible. Others argued for maximizing patient survival. Perhaps recognizing that the analysis of policy alternatives often makes the available trade-offs among relevant goals clear, some members argued for delaying the specification of goals until KPSAM could be used to begin to assess the consequences of alternative allocation rules. Although the discussion revealed a lack of consensus about the need for fundamental change, an in-depth review of current kidney allocation policy was set out as a committee goal at its July meeting.

In June 2004 the board directed the OPTN executive committee to coordinate a retreat in concert with the KTC to consider the concept of net benefit in kidney allocation policy. The retreat, which involved members of the executive committee and the KTC as well as other invited participants, was held in September. Concerned about the perceived problems of the allocation system, especially in light of the requirements of the Final Rule to seek equitable and best use of donated organs, the executive committee, in conjunction with the new chair of the KTC, Mayo Clinic transplant surgeon Mark Stegall, created the Kidney Allocation Review Subcommittee (KARS). The KARS would be a subcommittee of the KTC augmented with some additional people who Stegall thought would be helpful for achieving its mission of completing a comprehensive review of the kidney allocation system.

The KTC itself remained split over the need for fundamental change, as it conveyed in its November 2004 report to the board of directors: "While the Committee recognizes the system needs improvement, some members stated kidneys are currently allocated within a very solid allocation system that only requires minor tweaks. Other members were enthusiastic about possible major modifications to the allocation system, but cautioned that drastic changes could lead to greater unexpected inequities" (29).

The KARS took a very public approach to its task. During 2005 it held eleven public hearings on specific topics: review of the current kidney allocation system, scope of ESRD, ethics, barriers to access, OPO issues, histocompatibility, patient issues, minority issues, specific biological issues, net benefit models, and transplantation in other countries. For example, the March hearings on patient and minority affairs, which this author observed, sought comments on the current system from transplant candidates and recipients as well as other interested parties. Morning presentations were made by six transplant candidates or recipients drawn from diverse backgrounds, followed by representatives of the National Kidney Foundation, the Polycystic Kidney Disease Foundation, and the National Minority Organ and Tissue Education Program. The afternoon focused on minority affairs issues, including concerns about minorities being disadvantaged through delayed placement on the transplantation list.

These hearings, which concluded in May, identified a number of problems with the current system: inefficiency in the use of kidneys from expanded criteria donors, leading to wasted organs; lack of predictability of when individual patients will receive kidneys, making it difficult to keep medical data for transplant candidates up to date; continued variability in access to transplantation based on blood group (and therefore race) and geography; inefficiency in allocating kidneys to sensitized patients; and the allocation of kidneys from younger donors to older recipients, so that recipients often outlived the kidneys they received (OPTN 2008b, 7–8). Information from the public hearings, as well as the analysis of data from the SRTR, led the KARS to conclude that the kidney allocation system does not adequately balance utility and justice.

During this process, the KARS was already beginning to consider maximization of net benefits as an allocation system goal. This effort was reinforced in October 2005 at the board of directors strategic planning meeting. One of the workgroups specifically considered the appropriate role in organ allocation of net benefits, which it defined as "incremental reduction of burden of disease of receiving a transplant compared to not receiving a transplant at that time" (OPTN 2005, 2). The workgroup argued that net benefit is a valid consideration in an organ allocation system, but that it should generally not be the only consideration. Most important, it concluded that, if the OPTN is asked to consider a change in any organ allocation system, then the net benefit of that change should be calculated. Focusing on net benefit was further legitimized by the goals set out by the Health Resources and Services Administration (HRSA), the HHS agency that over-sees the OPTN and organ transplantation, through its Program Assessment Rating Tool exercise, a Bush administration initiative to facilitate performance budgeting (Gilmour and Lewis 2006). One of its goals was to increase the average number of life-years gained by recipients of deceased-donor kidneys.

During 2006 the KARS began to make progress in developing a concrete proposal for implementing net benefits. Two subcommittees were particularly important. The Variable Definitions Subcommittee worked to identify data for measuring relevant variables to be used in the allocation system that would be objective and not easily vulnerable to gaming. For example, what should determine if a patient is diabetic? The subcommittee rejected the commonly used fasting glucose test as a basis for definition because it could easily be gamed through changing the patient's diet. Instead, it selected a hemoglobin test that was less susceptible to manipulation. The Net Lifetime Survival Benefit Modeling Subcommittee focused on the choice of variables and methods to be used in predicting the net benefit for patients on the waiting list. As these efforts moved forward, the KARS continued to consider other factors potentially relevant to kidney allocation. For instance, the Hopefulness Subcommittee considered the implications of loss of hope of receiving transplants among those with low net benefit scores and the possibility of restoring hope by randomly allocating some fraction of kidneys. KARS members were also encouraged to propose alternatives to allocation based primarily on net benefits. Elements of some of these alternatives eventually found their way into the proposal that ultimately emerged. For example, Peter Stock, the KARS vice chair and later KTC chair, suggested allocating higher quality kidneys to patients with longer expected quality-adjusted gains in life-years and in placing some weight on time since the initiation of dialysis.

In February 2007 the KARS sought feedback on its efforts from the larger transplant community in a public forum held in Dallas, Texas. More than five hundred people participated in person or by conference call. Presentations in the morning session reviewed the shortcomings of the current allocation system, ethical considerations, and, most important, introduced life-years from transplant (LYFT) as the basis for implementing the net benefit principle. LYFT is the number of additional years any particular transplant candidate would be expected to gain from receiving a transplant. It is based on estimates of the candidate's median survival time with and without a transplant. These estimates were made using data from more than 110,000 people on the kidney transplant waiting list from 1992 through 2004, statistically accounting for the censoring of data for those with or without transplants who survived beyond 2004. The afternoon session included public testimony and group discussions.

The LYFT approach received generally favorable responses. Participants raised a number of concerns, however. Some feared that the proposal might have a negative impact on live donation. Relatively young patients, who often have more potential donors, including parents and other living relatives, would be more likely to have high LYFT scores and might therefore decide to wait for cadaveric kidneys rather than seek out live donors. Many participants believed that the dichotomous categorization of kidneys as from either standard criteria donors or extended kidney donors (see chapter 4), should be replaced with a continuous scale. A number of participants also urged the KARS to provide a careful transition plan that would not disadvantage candidates currently on the waiting list.

In August 2007 the KTC explicitly compared six allocation systems: first, the current system, which was assessed as inefficient, and in some ways, inequitable; second, a system based only on LYFT; third, a system that modifies LYFT scores using time on dialysis and the donor profile index (DPI), a continuous measure of the quality of donated kidneys; fourth, a system that divides donated organs into DPI quintiles and patients into LYFT quintiles and then matched the quintiles with priority given to patients within quintiles by time on dialysis; fifth, a system based on DPI quintiles and posttransplant survival quintiles, rather than LYFT quintiles; and, sixth, a system that matches organs to patients based only on age. The last two systems were rejected from further consideration: the fifth because it would offer fewer total life-years than any of the others, and the sixth because it would be unfair to older patients given that donors tended to be younger. After assessing the allocation systems in terms of average extra years of life, average posttransplant lifetime, and average graft lifetime, the committee decided to move forward with development of the third system, the modified LYFT system. In subsequent months, the committee received feedback on the proposal from several other committees: the Patient Affairs Committee, which asked whether the LYFT score could be modified to provide an incentive for patients to improve overall health, such as through weight loss; the Minority Affairs Committee, which asked that the effort consider geographic disparities; and the Ethics Committee, which stressed the importance of the system not discriminating in terms of age, race, or disease, and not reducing living donor transplants. The committee also received comments from the American Diabetes Association and the American Society of Transplantation.

At its December meeting the KTC took a number of votes that cleared the way for the preparation of a proposal that could be sent out for public comment. For example, the committee voted 19 to 11 with 1 abstention to cap the weight placed on LYFT scores to 80 percent to address the concern that those with high LYFT scores would not seek live donors. The committee planned to complete the concept proposal by February 2008 so that it could be presented at regional and committee meetings and to patient and professional organizations. Based on the feedback that resulted, it expected to revise the proposal and send it out for public comment during the summer of 2008 so that the board of directors could consider it at its November 2008 meeting.

In early 2008 the KARS did indeed complete the concept proposal, meeting by conference call almost weekly. The KTC presented the proposal to the board of directors in February. Although the KTC was prepared to vote to release the proposal for public review, it found itself in a procedural bind. Staff at the HRSA, which administers the OPTN and SRTR contracts, had some concern that the proposal might be challenged on the basis of age discrimination because age is one of the factors used in the estimation of LYFT scores. In an effort to head off such a challenge, members of the staff briefed the HHS Office of Civil Rights in November 2007. As of the March 2008 meeting of the KTC, the Office of Civil Rights had not issued a legal opinion or otherwise signaled approval. Some members of the KTC favored seeking feedback and moving forward even without an Office of Civil Rights opinion, but ultimately the committee decided to wait for the opinion. The author observed a certain frustration at the meeting among some of those who had worked on the nearly four-year development of the proposal.

Still without an opinion from the Office of Civil Rights in September 2008, the Kidney Transplantation Committee issued a "request for information" (OPTN 2008a). It posed specific questions seeking information on the advantages and limitations of the LYFT, DPI, and dialysis-time concepts, as well as solutions to any of the limitations identified by those offering comments. Rather than seeking comments on the earlier proposal, it sought detailed comments on the elements that would likely be in the final proposal. The three months given for responses allowed consideration to move forward while waiting for a legal opinion.

In January 2009 the KTC held a public forum on the elements of the proposal in St. Louis, Missouri. Approximately two hundred people participated. No clear and specific alternative concepts emerged, but participants made a number of suggestions about alternative ways of implementing the concepts. The committee decided to explore these suggestions through additional modeling before finalizing a proposal.

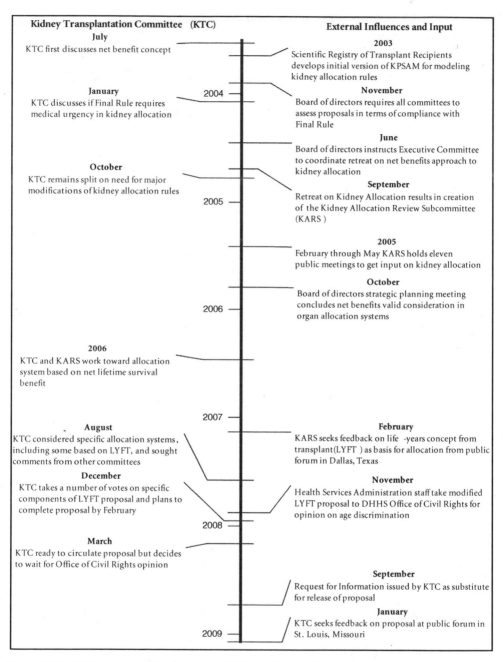

Kidney Transplantation Committee (KTC)

July
KTC first discusses net benefit concept

January
KTC discusses if Final Rule requires medical urgency in kidney allocation

October
KTC remains split on need for major modifications of kidney allocation rules

2006
KTC and KARS work toward allocation system based on net lifetime survival benefit

August
KTC considered specific allocation systems, including some based on LYFT, and sought comments from other committees

December
KTC takes a number of votes on specific components of LYFT proposal and plans to complete proposal by February

March
KTC ready to circulate proposal but decides to wait for Office of Civil Rights opinion

External Influences and Input

2003
Scientific Registry of Transplant Recipients develops initial version of KPSAM for modeling kidney allocation rules

November
Board of directors requires all committees to assess proposals in terms of compliance with Final Rule

June
Board of directors instructs Executive Committee to coordinate retreat on net benefits approach to kidney allocation

September
Retreat on Kidney Allocation results in creation of the Kidney Allocation Review Subcommittee (KARS)

2005
February through May KARS holds eleven public meetings to get input on kidney allocation

October
Board of directors strategic planning meeting concludes net benefits valid consideration in organ allocation systems

February
KARS seeks feedback on life-years concept from transplant(LYFT) as basis for allocation from public forum in Dallas, Texas

November
Health Services Administration staff take modified LYFT proposal to DHHS Office of Civil Rights for opinion on age discrimination

September
Request for Information issued by KTC as substitute for release of proposal

January
KTC seeks feedback on proposal at public forum in St. Louis, Missouri

2004
2005
2006
2007
2008
2009

Figure 7–1   Major Events in Development of Kidney Allocation Proposal

The time line shown in figure 7–1 summarizes this brief chronology. The left side of the figure shows major events within the kidney committee; the right side shows major external events. The time line ends with the public forum held in January 2009.

Components of the Kidney Allocation Score Proposal

The proposal gives the highest priority for any available cadaveric kidney to the patient on the local waiting list with the highest kidney allocation score (KAS) who is a candidate for a kidney-alone transplant. (Kidneys that are part of simultaneous kidney-pancreas, kidney-liver, or kidney-heart transplants would be allocated according to priority for those organs.) As shown in table 7–2, KAS depends on LYFT as well as the donor profile index, time on dialysis (DT), and the calculated panel reactive antibody (CPRA), a measure of sensitization. In addition to KAS, the proposed system would preserve the current pediatric and prior living donor priorities, limit mandatory sharing of zero-antigen mismatches to highly sensitized adult patients, incorporate the currently voluntary A_2/A_2B system, and phase out alternative allocation systems except for experimental purposes.

Definition and prediction of LYFT. The heart of the proposal is the introduction of LYFT as the starting point for allocation. The LYFT as defined in the proposal reflects three major decisions. First, a metric for predicting the number of years a patient would live with and without a transplant had to be selected. One possible choice was the average time of survival for some period, the approach used in lung allocation. However, the measure proved unstable when looking over the fifteen years needed to capture approximately 95 percent of patients without transplants and the 75 percent with transplants. Instead, median years of survival was chosen for its relative stability in the statistical analysis, which used Cox hazard models to estimate survival curves for those with and without transplants.

Second, variables for explaining survival in the hazard models had to be selected. Aside from the obvious requirements that the variables make statistically significant and clinically important contributions to explaining survival, the selected variables also are objective enough and measured with enough accuracy to avoid gaming and not raise ethical concerns. For example, race and primary insurance status were excluded for ethical reasons. Race was also excluded because, absent objective criteria, it could be selected by patients to increase their LYFT scores. The proposal uses the following variables: candidate age at offer, zero antigen mismatch, degree of mismatch on the HLA-DR loci, candidate local to donor, donor after cardiac death, donor age, donor cause of death, donor cytomegalovirus (CMV) serology, donor hypertension, donor weight, candidate years on dialysis at offer, candidate body mass index, candidate albumin level, candidate diabetes status, candidate with previous transplant, candidate CPRA, and candidate diagnosis of polycystic disease. The inclusion of age, which aside from pediatric priority does not appear in any of the other organ allocation systems, may be one of the reasons for the Office of Civil Rights review of the proposal.

Third, as quality of life generally improves substantially for those who receive transplants that result in functioning grafts, using quality-adjusted life-years rather than life-years as the underlying basis for LYFT was eventually viewed by KTC members as

Table 7–2   2008 Kidney Allocation Score Proposal

Kidney allocation score (KAS)
KAS = LYFT*0.8*(1–DPI) + DT*(0.8*DPI + 0.2) + (CPRA*4/100)
LYFT: life-years from transplant (candidate's median expected life span with a transplant from a specific available donor minus that candidate's utility-adjusted median projected wait-list survival without any transplant; both time after graft failure and time on dialysis weighted by a utility score of 0.80). Variables used to estimate LYFT: candidate age at offer, zero antigen mismatch, degree of mismatch on the HLA-DR loci, candidate local to donor, donor after cardiac death, donor age, donor cause of death, donor cytomegalovirus (CMV) serology, donor hypertension, donor weight, candidate years on dialysis at offer, candidate body mass index, candidate albumin level, candidate diabetes status, candidate previous transplant, candidate CPRA, candidate diagnosis of polycystic disease
DPI: donor profile index (continuous measure of donor organ viability: donor organs with longest survival potential assigned value of zero; donor organs with the shortest survival assigned a value of one). Variables used to estimate DPI: age, gender, race, height, weight, creatinine level, history of smoking, cardiac verus brain death, extended category donor under current definition, hepatitis C virus, history of hypertension, history of diabetes, and cause of death (anoxia, stroke, central nervous system tumor, other)
DT: dialysis time (years on dialysis)
CPRA: calculated panel reactive antibody (percentage of donors having one or more human leukocyte antigens considered incompatible or contraindicated for the transplant candidate)
Other features
Pediatric priority: continue to give those listed before age eighteen priority for kidneys from donors under thirty-five; continue to give those listed before age eighteen priority for zero mismatched kidneys; separate pediatric patients and adult candidates with pediatric candidates listed ahead of adult candidates at local, regional, and national levels for donors under thirty-five years.
Living donor priority: those who have made living organ donations continue to receive additional points as under current system
Zero-antigen mismatches: consideration of all (national or regional) highly sensitized adults (CPRA ≥ 80 percent) as adult local candidates; elimination of payback category
A_2 or A_2B donors: make mandatory current voluntary system allowing kidneys from blood type A_2 or A_2B donors to be transplanted into blood type B recipients
Variances: phase-out alternative allocation systems except for experimental purposes; review use of alternative allocation units

Source: Author's compilation based on OPTN/UNOS 2008.

appropriate. On the advice of SRTR analysts, and supported by the Scientific and Technical Advisory Committee, the KTC selected a utility weight of 0.80 to apply to years on dialysis, whether resulting from the patient not receiving a transplant or form post-transplant graft failure before death.

KAS versus pure LYFT.   Over the course of the development of the proposal, SRTR analysts simulated dozens of alternatives to the current policy using KPSAM. Simulations were based on the actual kidney transplant candidates and donated cadaveric kidneys for 2003. A variety of outcomes were assessed for each alternative, including total extra life-years, which is the most direct measure of net gain. Table 7–3 summarizes relevant outcomes resulting from three of the alternatives: the current system, allocation for standard criteria kidneys based purely on LYFT scores, and the KAS proposal. Note that the pure LYFT system greatly increases the total years after transplant, the total graft years, and the total extra life-years relative to the current system. For example, the pure LYFT system would increase the total number of life-years by 24 percent over the current system. In comparison, the KAS proposal increases the number by only 7 percent.

Why did the KTC choose the KAS proposal over the pure LYFT system? The KAS proposal evolved through a series of modifications made to address distributional concerns. One of these concerns was access to transplants for highly sensitized patients. As shown in table 7–3, moving from the current system to a pure LYFT system would dramatically reduce the proportion of highly sensitized patients (PRA ≥ 80) who received transplants from 13 percent to 5 percent and the proportion of the oldest patients (sixty-five and older) who received transplants from 12 percent to 6 percent. It would also offer only a negligible increase in the percent of African Americans receiving transplants. The additional components added to the KAS proposal trade off a substantial fraction of the net benefits gain that would be realized from the pure LYFT system to avoid penalizing highly sensitized patients and, as discussed below, to avoid creating a disincentive for live donation. These modifications also help address racial disparity and retain more of the current access for the oldest patients.

DPI.   The distinction between standard criteria donor and expanded criteria donor (ECD) kidneys complicates the current allocation system, imperfectly conveys kidney quality, and contributes to wasted organs though the pejorative connotations it places on ECD kidneys. The KAS proposal eliminates this dichotomous distinction, replacing it with the donor profile index, a continuous index of donor organ viability scaled to fall between zero and one. The estimation of DPI is based on the outcome of all adult kidney-alone transplants with deceased donor kidneys done from 1995 through 2005. The explanatory variables include donor age, gender, race, height, weight, creatinine level, smoking history, cardiac versus brain death, current ECD definition, presence of hepatitis C virus, history of hypertension, history of diabetes, and cause of death. The model predicts the probability of graft success for each donated kidney and these probabilities are transformed to a scale in which kidneys with the highest probability of graft survival have a score of zero and those with the lowest probability of graft survival have a score of one.

Table 7–3   Comparison of Alternative Allocation Rules

	Current system	Pure LYFT for SCD kidneys	KAS proposal
Total years after transplant	107,865	143,505	118,133
Total graft years	72,814	86,614	73,772
Total extra life-years	48,187	59,691	51,589
Percent increase in total years after transplant relative to current system	—	33	10
Percent increase in total graft years relative to current system	—	19	1
Percent increase in total extra life-years relative to current system	—	24	7
Percent of transplants to African Americans (36 percent of waiting list)	33	34	38
Percent of transplants to patients with PRA ≥ 80 (7 percent of waiting list)	13	5	14
Percent of transplants to patients 65 years and older (12 percent of waiting list)	12	6	9

Source: Author's compilation based on SRTR 2008.

The introduction of DPI allows all cadaveric kidneys to be allocated within a single system. As a continuous measure that can be used to adjust the weight placed on time on dialysis, it provides a lever through which relatively low quality kidneys can be allocated to those with small LYFT scores and long waiting times.

Dialysis time.   The KPSAM simulations assume that patients do not change their behavior related to their search for live donors. If patients with very high LYFT scores, often younger patients with relatively good chances of finding live donors, reduce their efforts to find live donors, then the full gains in net benefit relative to the current allocation system reported in the KPSAM simulations will not be realized in practice. To counter this possibility, the KAS proposal places some weight on the time patients have been on dialysis, reducing somewhat the priority of those with the highest LYFT scores. The lower scores imply somewhat longer expected waits for cadaveric organs and hence blunt the disincentive to search for a live donor.

After experimentation with a variety of weights, the KTC voted to distribute the weight between LYFT and time on dialysis such that the latter had at least 20 percent. So, for example, looking at the KAS equation in table 7–2, one sees that for the highest quality kidney (DPI equals 0) the minimum 20 percent of weight falls on dialysis time. As kidney quality falls (DPI greater than 0), the weight on dialysis time increases, so that for the poorest quality kidneys (DPI equals 0) 100 percent of the weight falls on dialysis time. There was no particular rationale for a minimum of 20 percent. Rather, it reflected both the concern about maintaining some incentive for the younger patients to seek live donors and the need to make a specific chose to move the design process forward.

As discussed in chapter 6, one of the incremental changes in kidney allocation supported by the KTC but rejected by the board of directors was the use of time from the initiation of dialysis rather than time on the kidney waiting list in the calculation of priority under the current system. The KAS proposal incorporates this incremental change desired by the Minority Affairs Committee and a majority of the KTC.

Calculated panel reactive antibody.   The current system gives four points to those with panel reactive antibody scores of 80 or greater. As shown in table 7–3, relying on LYFT scores alone would dramatically reduce the fraction of kidneys going to these highly sensitized patients. Including the term involving CPRA in the KAS proposal is intended to provide access to transplants for highly sensitized patients comparable to that under the current system.

During development of the KAS proposal, the Histocompatibility Committee, as noted in chapter 6, was working to replace panel reactive antibody (PRA) with CPRA. It advocated that this change be incorporated in the proposal. Because CPRA is on a scale of 0 to 100, it is converted to a fraction by dividing by 100. The result is then multiplied by 4 so that highly sensitized patients, those with CPRAs between 80 and 100, would receive points that ranged from 3.2 to 4. The discontinuity of the current system would be eliminated by giving less sensitized patients points based on their level of sensitization. Because the current system and the KAS proposal differ in the way they allocate points aside from sensitization, it is not necessarily the case that awarding approximately as many points to highly sensitized patients in each system would result in similar outcomes. Nonetheless, as shown in table 7–3, this appears to be the consequence.

Other components.   The KAS proposal preserves the priority given to patients listed by age eighteen for kidneys from deceased donors under thirty-five years old. It also preserves the priority given to patients who were previously organ donors. The mandatory national sharing of kidneys for whom there is a patient with zero-antigen mismatches is eliminated along with the associated payback requirements. However, a highly sensitized patient with zero-antigen mismatches is treated as if he or she were on the local waiting list. That is, if his or her KAS is larger than that of any local candidate, he or she is offered the kidney. The A_2/A_2B voluntary system is mandatory under the proposal. Finally, the proposal eliminates the use of alternative allocation systems except for experimental purposes.

The dog that didn't bark: Geography.   Although the KARS received a number of comments along the way urging a change in the current geographic basis of kidney allocation— priority first locally, then regionally, and finally nationally—the KAS proposal preserves it. There are several explanations. First, and probably most important, substantially changing the geographic basis of kidney allocation would have been politically difficult. Controversy over reducing the role of geography would likely have doomed the larger proposal that included it. Were the KAS proposal adopted, it would be natural to reconsider geography within its context. Second, there are real substantive concerns about the impact that broader geographic allocation would have on organ procurement. As discussed in chapter 4, effective procurement of organs depends on the efforts of transplant surgeons. Making cadaveric kidneys even more of a common property resource risks reducing the willingness of surgeons to make these efforts. As with the concern about the impact of the KAS proposal on live donation, the impact of changes in the allocation system on procuring cadaveric organs is beyond the capacity of the KPSAM model. Third, realistically assessing the consequences of broader geographic sharing would require modifying the KPSAM model to take account of cold ischemic times in predicting graft success. Thus, both political and analytical limitations led to a KAS proposal to keep the current geographic basis of allocation.

Patterns of Organizational Interaction

The development of the KAS proposal was spearheaded by the KARS and shepherded toward completion by the KTC. Nonetheless, throughout the process there was a close working relationship with the SRTR, extensive consultation with other OPTN committees, and solicitation of feedback from the transplant community. The broad pattern of this interaction is sketched in figure 7–2. Although the figure may appear complex, it grossly simplifies the interactions. For example, HRSA has ex officio members on all committees, suggesting the need for arrows from HRSA to each committee. Committee memberships overlap, with some people serving on more than one committee and many committees having designated representatives on other committees, suggesting that the boxes for committees should be shown as overlapping and more densely connected. Each committee reports regularly to the board of directors, which often directs committees to take up tasks, suggesting the need for arrows connecting the board with each committee. The SRTR does analysis supporting the efforts of many of the committees, suggesting another set of arrows. Committees and their members interact with the broader transplant community, suggesting yet another set of arrows. Comprehensively taking account of all these interactions would result in a very rich but incomprehensible figure.

Rather than comprehensively tracing the various intra- and interorganizational interactions, it is more valuable to assess qualitatively how well they allowed for the integration of evidence, expertise, and values. The assessment requires an answer to the question, compared to what? As with the assessment of the evolution of liver allocation rules at the end of chapter 5, it is useful to contrast the development of the KAS proposal with public rulemaking, the most likely alternative form of governance for transplantation policy in the United States.

The most striking contrast between the KAS proposal development and public rulemaking is transparency. Most public rulemaking reveals itself through two publications in the *Federal Register*: the proposed and the final rulemaking. Scholars have paid little attention to the informal processes of communication with interest groups and intra-

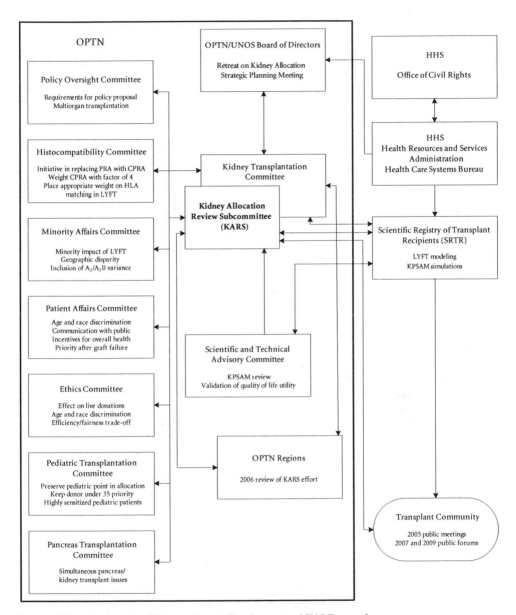

Figure 7–2   Organizational Interactions in Development of KAS Proposal

agency analysis and consultation that goes on during the drafting of proposals (West 2005). Indeed, no data are available for estimating how long on average this process takes, and the lack of transparency hinders the study of rule development. In contrast, the OPTN rule development process is amazingly open. Almost all of the substantive work is done within committees that hold meetings open to the public. Summaries of the discussions and votes of the committees are generally available in reports to the board of directors that are posted on the OPTN website. Although the accessibility of this material could be improved—through more complete electronic archiving and a better search engine for the OPTN website as well as the posting of the analytical reports supporting OPTN committees on the SRTR website—it is enough to allow anyone with an interest in a particular issue to follow the development of policies related to it. In the case of the KAS proposal, efforts were also made to engage the broader transplant community through public meetings and forums.

Another difference is the level of engagement of stakeholders in the development of rules. As noted, we know very little about the general role of interests in the development of proposed rules by agencies. We know somewhat more about the impacts of interest groups on the content of final rules. For example, a study of forty randomly selected routine rules issued by four federal agencies found that business interests, but not other interests, influenced the content of final rules through comments on proposed rules (Yackee and Yackee 2006). As discussed in chapter 2, we also know that agencies seek to engage stakeholders with desired expertise through advisory committees, but we have little systematic evidence of the influence of these committees on the content of rules. In contrast, stakeholders directly developed the KAS proposal. The most directly relevant expertise was provided by the members of the KTC. The sources of expertise were further extended through the addition of non-KTC members to the KARS. Throughout the development process, the chairs and other members of the KARS and the KTC met with other committees, whose members offered somewhat different expertise, to brief them on the development of the proposal and receive feedback. These consultations resulted in many substantive changes to the original LYFT proposal. Based on the additional information provided by the September 2008 request for information and the January 2009 forum, and absent a negative opinion by the Office of Civil Rights, the proposal will be fully specified in detail, issued for public comment like a proposed public rule, and, finally, after responses are made to the public comments, submitted to the board of directors for a formal vote.

Conclusion

The development of the KAS proposal shows that the process that permits frequent incremental adjustments in OPTN policies can also be used to formulate and assess policy alternatives involving fundamental change. The lead committee, in this case the KTC, serves as a locus for bringing together systematic evidence, appropriate modeling, tacit knowledge, and values. The intercommittee consultation further expands the sources of relevant expertise, reveals interests, and raises values. Votes within the committee allow decisions to be made that move the policy development forward even in the absence of a consensus. In other words, the OPTN seems to provide an attractive model of governance for implementing evidence-based medicine in the face of scarcity with immediate life and death consequences. The next chapter offers a more comprehensive assessment of OPTN performance and sets the stage for answering, in the final chapter, the question of whether the OPTN form of governance is sui generis or applicable in other medical contexts.

8

━━━━━○◆○━━━━━

How and How Well
Does the OPTN Govern?

Like zoologists sizing up unfamiliar animals, the previous chapters in this volume have tried to put the OPTN into an appropriate and useful category and then to observe its operations to understand how it functions in its environment. Whereas zoologists generally do not concern themselves with normative questions about the goodness of the animal in its niche, we want to know if the OPTN governs well. Doing so requires, first, an overall assessment of how the OPTN produces and administers policy, and, second, an evaluation of the extent to which these policies promote appropriate social goals. Completing these tasks sets the stage for hypothesizing, which I do in the final chapter, about the conditions under which a private rulemaker like the OPTN should be considered an institutional alternative for medical governance and the features of the OPTN that contribute to desirable outcomes.

The assessment of the outcomes poses a methodological challenge. Ideally, one would identify many governance institutions, including private rulemakers, dealing with the same or at least similar issues. With large enough numbers, one could assess possible systematic differences in outcomes between private rulemakers and other institutional forms statistically. With especially rich data that included private rulemakers with some variation in their forms, one might even be able to make inferences about the importance of particular institutional features. Unfortunately, we do not have such natural variation in institutional forms. Indeed, despite the efforts in chapter 2 to identify other institutions of medical governance that share features of private rulemaking, we really have but a single case if we take the institution as the unit of analysis.

Of course, case studies of single institutions or particular historical episodes have made fundamentally important contributions to the way we think about public administration and public policy. Philip Selznick's account of the Tennessee Valley Authority (1949), Herbert Kaufman's focus on the norms of rangers in the Forest Service (1960), Graham Allison's multiple interpretations of the Cuban Missile Crisis (1971), and Jeffrey Pressman and Aaron Wildavsky's tale of the implementation of federal programs in Oakland (1973) are just some of the more prominent examples of influential case studies. Ultimately, however, these great successes in presenting general ideas about how the world works require us to rely very heavily on the authors' interpretations of empirical evidence arising in fairly narrow and potentially idiosyncratic contexts.

The challenge of making effective use of case studies often confronts international relations researchers who wish to take advantage of specific events that provide windows into otherwise opaque decision-making processes, and comparative politics researchers who can confidently compare only a small number of countries because of the large investments required to understand national contexts adequately and gather relevant empirical evidence. In recent years, scholars in these fields have become more methodologically self-conscious about how to design effective case studies (George and Bennett 2005). In-depth case studies offer the possibility of discovering the causal mechanisms linking exogenous causes to outcomes, thereby providing evidence relevant to the assessment of the validity of the hypothesized relationship between cause and effect. For an overview and discussion of the multiple interpretations of causal mechanisms, see Gerring 2008. They also provide a basis for the inductive development of theory. When the case studies take a narrative form, guided by either explicit or implicit hypotheses about the behavior being studied, they are called process tracing (George and Bennett 2005).

The previous five chapters offer six narratives on the OPTN and its policymaking. The narrative in chapter 3 simply explains the conversion of the OPTN from a voluntary network to a formal network with authority to act as a private rulemaker. The next four chapters look in detail at the factors contributing to decision making within this private rulemaker. This process tracing considers five narratives: explicating the origins and evolution of policies related to organ supply, the extended controversy over the geographic basis of liver allocation, the response to concerns about racial disparity in kidney allocation, the nonincremental change in lung allocation rules, and the attempted nonincremental change in kidney allocation rules. Kidneys and livers are the most important transplant organs, in terms of numbers, aggregate costs, and public concerns. Because the narratives of the development of allocation rules for these two organs span most of the OPTN history, they provide an appropriate basis for an overall assessment of its decision making. To the extent that the narratives display similar decision-making processes, one can be more confident in characterizing OPTN decision making in general.

Here I draw on these narratives to investigate a number of hypotheses suggested by the comparison of public and private rulemaking in chapter 2. In the next and concluding chapter, I draw on them to hypothesize about the features of the OPTN that contribute to the observed outcomes and the extent to which institutions with these features should be considered as possible alternatives for medical governance.

Incremental Rather Than Episodic Rulemaking

Building on the work of economic historian Brian Arthur (1994), political scientists have argued that economies of scale create path dependence in policy making (Pierson 2000). As Scott Page noted, a variety of externalities can lead to past policies influencing the choice of future policies (2006). Although changes in rules for the allocation of cadaveric organs are not strictly zero sum—the number of successfully transplanted patients can be expanded by rules that contribute to higher rates of graft success or to more effective procurement of organs—these changes usually involve strong negative externalities in that increasing access for one group necessarily reduces access for other groups. The greater psychological saliency of losses over gains (Kahneman and Tversky 1984), as well as the greater ease with which small numbers of potential losers relative to large numbers of potential gainers can overcome the collective action problem, suggest the important influence of current on future policy—what Page would call state dependence rather than path dependence. Rolling the process back to the initial policy, one might reasonably predict policy stasis. In other words, a plausible hypothesis would be that the initial rules would not change absent some scandal or other crisis that opened a policy window during which potential gainers from change could be mobilized to counter the potential losers, within either the institution or the political system within which it operates.

Yet, as noted in chapter 2, based on comparisons across a number of well-matched case studies, Ross Cheit contrasted the episodic adoption of product standards by public agencies with the "prospective and ongoing" incremental adjustment of standards by private standard-setters (1990, 202). Although one might not necessarily expect this characterization to hold when choosing zero-sum allocation rules rather than standards that, at least initially, are voluntary, the most general hypothesis is that decision making within the OPTN, a private rulemaker, involves more frequent and incremental adjustments than would be the case if HHS were making the rules. All we know about traditional regulation suggests that HHS would not make frequent adjustments. Consequently, frequent rule changes by the OPTN would support the assessment that, at least in this context, private rulemaking yields different patterns of decision making than public rulemaking would.

Turning to the narratives, it is clear that the policies the OPTN initially adopted did indeed influence the policies in place two decades later. Most obviously, the priority for allocating locally procured organs to local patients, which originated in the voluntary sharing that preceded the OPTN, remains important in the allocation rules for kidneys, livers, and lungs. Further, human leucocyte antigen (HLA) matching, which was very important in the initial kidney allocation policy, has been only gradually reduced in importance. With respect to organ procurement, the strong preference for brain-death donors at the time the OPTN was created made cardiac-death donations exceptional within the allocation rules. Also, the decision by the Task Force on Organ Transplantation to emphasize the importance of giving donor families the opportunity to act altruistically legitimized the customary practice that procurement personnel ignore the expressed intention to donate unless it is supported by the next of kin.

Nonetheless, an evolution of rules in each of these areas is evident. The incremental response to concerns about racial disparity in kidney allocation is the clearest case. In 1995 and 2003 substantial reductions were made in the weight given to HLA matching. A number of changes have also been made in the rules governing mandatory sharing of zero-HLA mismatched kidneys nationally. Further, the Minority Affairs Committee was especially influential in initiating a voluntary variance to allow allocating A_2 and A_2B kidneys to patients with type B or O blood, which by 2007 had been adopted by almost a fifth of the organ procurement organizations. The effort by the Kidney and Pancreas Transplantation Committee to base waiting time on the initiation of dialysis rather than the time of addition to the waiting list proved much more controversial; its committee-sponsored variance has not yet attracted wide participation from organ procurement organizations.

The initiative to make fundamental change in kidney allocation policy, which has been under way since 2005, might raise some question about the incremental nature of OPTN policymaking if it is eventually adopted. However, it is interesting that decision making during gestation of the fundamental change, introducing net benefit as a primary allocation goal, was itself incremental. The plan on the table changed in steps from one that placed full weight on net benefit to one that restored some weight on waiting time and sensitivity and that builds in an incentive to accept organs from less desirable donors. The same incremental process in the development of a fundamentally different allocation system was apparent in the successful effort between 1999 and 2005 to introduce a lung allocation system that placed weight on short-run net benefit as well as waiting time. In other words, it is possible for the OPTN incremental process, with its extensive consultation and committee votes to propel it forward, to produce nonincremental change.

The allocation rules for livers underwent small but frequent changes before, during, and after the Final Rule controversy. Before the controversy, the imminent death category was eliminated because of its abuse by some transplant centers; the number of priority categories was reduced; points for waiting time were adjusted; and local priority was redefined to include all transplant centers served by the organ procurement organization that retrieved the liver. A number of changes were made to build confidence in the integrity of patient classification in anticipation of moving to regional sharing. One of these changes, redefining the highest priority group to include only patients with acute liver failure, provided the opening for advocates of wider geographic allocation to take the issue public when the OPTN rejected committee recommendations to move to regional allocation. During the almost four years of the controversy, regional review boards were created to audit status assignments, separate medical urgency criteria were set for pediatric patients, and more objective scoring systems were introduced to assess the severity of illness of adult and then of pediatric patients and to establish priority for the sickest patients in the region over less ill local patients. After the controversy, small adjustments continued to be made to the new allocation system.

One of the more significant changes after the controversy was the elimination of payback provisions—a balancing of transfers among organ procurement organizations over time. Regional allocation for the highest priority patients was initially implemented through alternative sharing arrangements that allowed several regions with concerns about the integrity of patient classification to limit their risks of exploitation. In 2005, with the integrity of patient classification established, the OPTN eliminated the use of paybacks in liver allocation.

Change in organ procurement has originated from a variety of sources, including initiatives by state and federal governments, private organizations, and OPTN member organizations. The OPTN itself has made a number of changes to allocation rules to expand the available pool of organs. For example, to encourage the use of donations following cardiac death, kidneys from such donors were exempted from national sharing for zero-HLA mismatches. Local waiting lists of patients willing to accept extended criteria kidneys (those from older and sicker donors) were established. Extended criteria kidneys not immediately claimed for patients with zero-HLA mismatches were made available to those on the waiting list according to waiting time. Subsequently, payback for the extended criteria donor kidneys shared nationally were eliminated to remove any disincentive for transplant centers to encourage patients to accept these kidneys.

The OPTN showed some reluctance to take a role in live donation, partly because responsibility for overseeing live donation was not explicitly set out in the National Organ Transplant Act. Nonetheless, the OPTN did approve variances to allow list exchange donations to enable people to add their donated kidneys to the cadaveric pool in return for cadaveric organs going to the patients they wished to help. After legal clarification, the OPTN began adopting standards for live donation. Somewhat behind regional activity, it also began putting in place a framework for facilitating nationwide paired exchanges.

The narratives in this volume thus show a consistent pattern of frequent incremental changes in policies. We can never know whether HHS rulemaking would have produced a similar pattern. However, based on what we know about public rulemaking in general, it seems unlikely that we would observe frequent incremental change for largely zero sum allocation rules. Instead, we should expect infrequent, but perhaps more substantial, change driven by exogenous events that allow the resistance of self-perceived losers to be overcome. Although caution is needed in making predictions about the behavior of the HHS in the absence of the OPTN from its behavior in the presence of the OPTN, the history of the Final Rule is at least consistent with the notion of episodic rather than frequent rulemaking. So too is the observation that the few de facto rules of the OPTN made de jure deal with data collection rather than allocation.

Use of Expertise

The desirability of evidence-based medicine has become a mantra among health policy researchers and advocates. However, as noted in chapter 1, in the United States the incorporation of more efficacious treatments into routine patient care lags their discovery on average by about fifteen to twenty years (Institute of Medicine 2001, 145). Indeed, one of the reasons that organizations like the Oregon Health Services Commission and National Institute for Health and Clinical Excellence in the United Kingdom have received so much attention from health policy experts is that they are viewed as exceptional in the application of evidence-based medicine. (The Advisory Committee on Immunization Practices also deserves attention for this reason.) In view of the dearth of identified governance arrangements for implementing evidence-based medicine expeditiously, it would not be surprising if OPTN decisions lacked a strong basis in medical evidence.

Yet, one of the reasons for the choice of private rulemaking in other contexts, such as agricultural marketing boards, the allocation of Internet domain names, and securities self-regulatory agencies, is the valuable tacit knowledge that stakeholders bring to the table (Weimer 2006). These private rulemakers do not necessarily have a relative advantage over their public counterparts in collecting or using data germane to assessing outcomes, an observation Cheit made in his comparison of private and public standard-setters (1990). However, the OPTN was created in tandem with the SRTR, an exceptionally comprehensive database in terms of both universal and longitudinal coverage. One may therefore hypothesize that the combination of tacit knowledge and the availability of data to support scientific investigation would give the OPTN great potential for applying evidence-based medicine.

The narratives show this potential being substantially realized over the entire history of the OPTN, and perhaps even more so after the Final Rule and the selection of a separate contractor to administer the SRTR. (Reliance on scientific evidence appears to have become greater and more sophisticated, but some of the increases may be due to improvements in data, particularly the accumulation over time of longer longitudinal coverage, and modeling capability that might have occurred regardless.) The evidence brought to bear includes not just scientific evidence of a statistical nature but also the tacit knowledge of stakeholders about likely behavioral responses to rule changes and other considerations that cannot be addressed by interrogating the available data.

Consider some of the uses of scientific evidence in the evolution of liver allocation rules. Simulation models based on the SRTR data supported the decision to limit the highest priority patient group to those suffering from acute liver disease by showing that these patients would suffer fewer graft failures requiring re-transplantation and thus result in a net increase in the number of lives saved. Both proponents and opponents of national sharing of livers used these models to support their cases, though these models did not show large differences in lives saved or life-years gained between the local-first status quo and national alternatives. Statistical modeling and verification were very important in developing and introducing the MELD/PELD system for classifying the severity of liver disease, an important preliminary step to regional sharing. Beyond these instances, committee reports and transcripts show a prominent role for analyses based on SRTR data. Most often these analyses were and are conducted by SRTR staff, usually at the request of the committee. The committees, however, also routinely considered analyses by independent researchers using the SRTR data.

The evolution of kidney allocation rules shows a similar pattern. Scientific evidence played a role in almost every discussion of rule changes. Documentation of longer waiting times for kidney transplants for African Americans set the stage for the series of changes in the weight placed on HLA matching. Studies showing declines in the importance of partial HLA matches for graft success changed the perceived trade-off between medical efficiency and social equity.

The initial variance to allow an organ procurement organization to transplant A_2 and A_2B kidneys to patients with type B and O blood was based on experiments done before the creation of the OPTN and analyses of results from the variance led to the participation of more organ procurement organizations. The definition of expanded criteria donor was based on statistical analyses to determine the factors that would raise the risk of graft failure by a specified amount above that for kidneys from donors meeting the standard criteria. Committee deliberations over kidney allocation rules, like those for liver allocation rules, have relied heavily on analyses and simulations based on SRTR data.

The proposal to include net benefit in kidney allocation shows the importance of analyses from the SRTR at every step of the process. The net benefit measure, life-years from transplant, depends on statistically sophisticated predictions of longevity following transplant with a specific kidney and longevity on the waiting list. Demonstrations that the underlying distributions of graft success for standard and extended donor kidneys overlapped led to a continuous donor profile index that could be used to integrate all donations into a unified allocation system that would create an incentive for more patients to accept kidneys from less preferred donors. The proposal also includes the more sophisticated approach to determining sensitivity developed by the Histocompatability Committee, which relied heavily on SRTR data analyses. The movement from a proposal based exclusively on net benefit to one that incorporated other factors was driven by simulations showing trade-offs between efficiency and distributional goals.

Although not as obvious as the role of scientific evidence, the tacit knowledge of stakeholders also influenced the policy development in important ways. First, transplant professionals often raised questions based on their experiences that could be investigated with SRTR data. In raising concerns about patients who might be disadvantaged by rule changes, for example, they contributed to a level of sophistication that would otherwise be difficult for analysts removed from clinical experience. Second, transplant professionals' clinical experiences also enabled them to anticipate behavioral responses to proposed rule changes. This shaped policy in a variety of ways. Some examples include an understanding of how qualitative classifications of patients could, and were, being manipulated propelled the move to quantitative classifications based on objective data for liver patients before moving to regional sharing and for lung patients as part of the new system of allocation based on net benefit; careful setting of default values for missing data in classification systems to reduce the opportunity for manipulation by delaying the provision of up-to-date data; and modification of the kidney allocation proposal to counter the reduced incentive that the emphasis on net benefits would provide for young patients to seek live donors.

Aside from the influence of scientific and tacit knowledge on allocation rules, one might also point to the continuous improvement and fairly rapid spread of transplant technology as evidence of successful evidence-based medicine. Some caution is needed, however, because rapid technological change characterized transplantation before the OPTN was created. The safer claim is therefore that the private rulemaking of the OPTN has not slowed the introduction and rapid diffusion of new technology.

The amount and technical sophistication of scientific evidence used in rulemaking appear to have increased somewhat since the Final Rule was promulgated and the administration of the OPTN and the SRTR separated. The former helped set higher expectations about the level of evidence needed to justify rule changes and made the possibility of reversal of rules by HHS somewhat more credible. The latter promoted some independence in establishing the analytic agenda. Overall, these changes probably further strengthened the already strong role of evidence-based medicine within the OPTN.

It is interesting that in the one prominent case in which the OPTN and HHS were in open dispute over scientific issues, the cold ischemic time for livers and the feasibility of national sharing, the Institute of Medicine assessment mandated by Congress largely supported the OPTN positions. HHS, of course, was disadvantaged in writing its proposed rules without the benefit of its own advisory committee system for organ transplantation.

Could expertise be as effectively tapped through public HHS rulemaking? Although it would be impractical for HHS to maintain cutting-edge transplantation expertise within its staff, the department would be able to establish advisory committees of the sort that it routinely uses in other policy areas. These committees would likely not be as effective in using expertise as the OPTN, however, for several reasons. First, applying the arguments of

Sheila Jasanoff (1990) and Bruce L. R. Smith (1992), expertise would likely be less effective if it were separated from the development of rules. Second, the weaker link to rulemaking would probably reduce the willingness of transplant professionals to share their expertise through committee service, in part because participating in votes that shape rules offers a greater sense of efficacy and is thus more rewarding than offering advice that may or may not have any impact. Third, achieving productive interaction across committees with distinct but related charges would be challenging within a federal advisory system geared toward individual advisory committees. Most likely, it would require joint meetings of relevant committees as is sometimes done by the Food and Drug Administration when there are broad issues. Fourth, conflict of interest issues would have to be addressed in a flexible way because the most relevant expertise is held by the stakeholders. Many advisory committees at HHS, such as its Medicare Evidence Development & Coverage Advisory Committee and the Food and Drug Administration's drug and device committees, provide for industry representation in membership but not in voting. Would a transplant surgeon be viewed as an expert and given a vote, or as an employee of a transplant center, part of the regulated industry, and not given a vote? Creating a system of advisory committees as effective as the OPTN in applying expertise to rule development would not be impossible, but it would be difficult.

Professional Norms and the Accommodation of Interests

Private rulemakers may be technically efficient in pursuing outcomes that do not promote social welfare. For example, agricultural marketing boards may effectively restrict supply to maximize rents for their members, but at the expense of consumers and perhaps society overall. The problem arises because important stakeholders, consumers of the good, either are absent from the table or have little influence relative to the more knowledgeable and self-interested producers. Assuming that those with the greatest expertise and strongest private interests will be the most influential participants, one might expect that the OPTN would be dominated by transplant professionals to the detriment of patient interests.

Indeed, the financial interests of the transplant physicians and their centers are particularly strong. As noted in chapter 4, transplantation is one of the more profitable types of surgery for hospitals (Resnick et al. 2005). Obtaining more of the scarcest resource needed for transplantation—cadaveric organs—generally translates into higher earnings for surgeons and larger profits for centers as well as often immense gratitude from their patients who receive successful grafts. Transplant surgeons thus have a strong incentive to seek rules that allocate more organs to their own patients.

At the same time, transplant professionals bring with them norms that may align their preferences more closely to the interests of patients than would otherwise be the case. The strongest of these norms for the physicians, who are most influential in the OPTN committees, is promoting the welfare of their patients. However, they also share norms about the desirability of promoting health and the fairness in the distribution of health care—observers note that, since creation of the OPTN, "references to justice and equitable access have become part of the everyday vocabulary of those involved with transplantation" (Benjamin, Cohen, and Grochowski 1994, 860)—as well as the appropriate use of evidence in assessing medical treatments, though they may bring with them differing perspectives that affect these assessments. Congress set expectations that these norms would be influential by charging the OPTN to employ medical criteria in matching patients with organs. Therefore, it is possible that, even in the presence of strong interests, their being consistent with or moderated by professional norms would tend to align technical efficiency with patient interests and other social values.

Conflicting interests among stakeholders was most apparent in controversy over the role of geography in liver allocation. A large transplant center led the effort to eliminate local priority in the face of opposition from many smaller centers, which dominated the board of directors, a majority rule body. Frustrated by the failure to eliminate local priority, especially when the board failed to adopt committee recommendations for regional sharing, the large center took the issue to the president and the secretary of HHS, setting off the Final Rule controversy. The smaller centers were able to mobilize support in Congress, partly because of their presence in many congressional districts but also because many members of Congress were skeptical about the desirability of HHS imposing rules on the transplant community. Indeed, most supporters of national sharing did not want the OPTN to lose its primary role in developing policy.

The self-interested positions of the transplant centers were consistent with the welfare of their own patients. Arguments could be made for both positions from the perspective of social welfare. On the one hand, somewhat broader sharing would better satisfy the value of medical need by getting more livers to the sickest patients. On the other, this would not likely maximize net benefit as measured by a metric like incremental life years. Further, broader sharing could reduce the effort invested by transplant centers in organ procurement. The move from local to regional sharing that actually occurred seems to be a reasonable compromise in terms of social values, though many of the participants would undoubtedly not characterize the process surrounding the change as reasonable.

Broad consultation, both within the OPTN and through solicitation of public comments, often brings to the fore interests beyond those of the transplant centers. Proposed rule changes frequently elicit comments from organizations representing those with specific diseases or patients on waiting lists concerned about their priority. For example, repeated proposals to calculate waiting time for kidneys in a way less disadvantageous to African Americans have been successfully opposed.

There may also be what might be called professional interests as well as professional values. For instance, debates over the importance of HLA matching in kidney allocation reflected to some extent the degree of investment various participants had made in the science of tissue typing. Those who pioneered tissue typing tended to require more evidence to be convinced that less weight could be put on HLA matching without sacrificing graft success. The reluctance of organ procurement personnel to place the wishes of the donor over those of the next of kin may reflect the difficulty of confronting grieving relatives as well as concerns about community support for donation.

Nonetheless, the Final Rule controversy aside, that narrow interest does not appear to be the primary force driving rulemaking in a policy area with literally life and death consequences is a surprising finding. One explanation is that often interests and professional norms coincide so that self-interested and patient-interested behavior are indistinguishable. Another may be that most of the professionals involved bring with them an understanding and commitment to reliance on scientific evidence, and the SRTR has made such evidence relatively abundant.

As argued in chapter 2, private rulemaking may be politically attractive for Congress in circumstances, such as the allocation of transplant organs, where the potential for blame exceeds the opportunity for credit claiming. The Final Rule controversy, in which HHS attempted to impose policy, forced the issue onto the congressional agenda, suggesting that had responsibility for the development of allocation rules been delegated to the HHS, Congress would be frequently drawn into policy disputes with their largely unfavorable balances of blame and credit. Rather than congressional involvement being exceptional, it would likely be routine. Had that been the case, the narratives presenting the evolution of liver and kidney allocation rules would almost certainly have revealed more conventional interest group politics. That they did not suggests that medical governance arrangements can affect the nature of the politics surrounding wicked problems. More broadly, the now trite claim that institutions matter appears valid.

Does the OPTN Produce Good Policy?

A full normative assessment of OPTN rulemaking would require specifying the possibly relevant social goals and, because any rule will almost certainly involve some conflict among these goals, establishing their relative importance. The current allocation rules for different organs emphasize different goals. For example, liver allocation seems consistent primarily with a version of medical efficiency defined in terms of avoiding immediate deaths. However, as with allocation rules for other organs, the priority given to pediatric over adult patients indirectly promotes the utilitarian goal of allocating organs so as to produce the largest aggregate gain in life-years. The current kidney allocation rules reflect trade-offs among several valid goals: weight on HLA matching to promote medical efficiency, in terms of maximizing graft success; weight for sensitized patients to promote medical justice, by giving these patients better chances of receiving transplants; and weight on waiting time to promote sociological justice, by giving greater access to African Americans and other patients otherwise disadvantaged by medically based allocation rules. The evolution of the proposal for a new kidney allocation system based on net benefit showed an initial utilitarian emphasis on maximizing life-years with subsequent modifications to give weight to medical justice (relative priority for sensitized patients), social justice (weight for waiting time to reduce racial disparity), and supply efficiency (incentives to accept less desirable organs and muting of disincentives for young patients to seek live donors).

Less demanding than assessing whether the rules place appropriate weights on these goals is to determine whether changes in rules reflect appropriate evidence-based and value-conscious deliberation. Evidence-based rulemaking is a prerequisite for technical efficiency in regulating any complex and rapidly changing activity. Being explicit about values is a prerequisite for technical efficiency to promote social goals.

This discussion makes a strong case that the OPTN's frequent and incremental rule changes are supported by extensive and appropriate use of data and tacit knowledge. In general, consideration of rule changes appear to arise in the context of better promoting appropriate values. Sometimes the concerns coincide with, and are therefore indistinguishable from, stakeholder interests; other times they arise without any clear connection to such interests, but rather stem from general concerns about efficiency or fairness. In comparison to the counterfactual of public regulation, the OPTN appears quite successful in achieving technical efficiency and promoting appropriate social values.

As argued in chapter 1, governance arrangements should also be assessed in terms of democratic accountability. On the one hand, the actual rulemaking process within the OPTN is as least as accountable as it is within the HHS. In addition to notice and comment procedures that parallel those used in public rulemaking, the development of rules within the OPTN is much more transparent and open—much of the work is done in open meetings with transcripts and recorded votes—than it is in federal agencies. On the other hand, the OPTN is less accountable to elected representatives than HHS is—the OPTN does not need annual appropriations from Congress; it elects its own officers, who are not subject to Senate approval, as are the highest ranked officers of executive agencies; and it is rarely subject to congressional oversight. Instead, the OPTN is accountable to the HHS secretary. Thus, electoral accountability is attenuated to some extent through HHS. Before the Final Rule, the extent to which HHS could influence OPTN rulemaking was ambiguous. After it, the nature of HHS oversight became clearer but remains indirect. HHS staff participate in OPTN meetings as ex officio members, but largely as observers. The OPTN de facto rules become de jure only when they are promulgated by the HHS secretary, who could block specific rules, but these are powers that influence the OPTN through their potential rather than actual application. The argued advantages that the OPTN enjoys in terms of technical efficiency and promotion of social values come at the expense of direct electoral accountability, but not necessarily at the expense of authentic public participation in rulemaking.

David Rosenbloom argues that when administrative units make rules they are engaged in legislative functions and thus serve as extensions of Congress (2000, 134). In the case of the OPTN, Congress effectively delegated a legislative function to a self-governing organization of its own creation. It subsequently allowed HHS to strengthen its oversight role and retain de jure authority over rulemaking. However, it also intervened during the Final Rule controversy with a moratorium to block the attempt by HHS to impose substantive content to allocation rules, and the House actually passed legislation that would have denied HHS its de jure authority altogether. One interpretation of the "legislative" role of the OPTN is that Congress chose an institutional arrangement that would engage stakeholders directly in rulemaking rather than indirectly through lobbying or involvement in a formal rulemaking process. Congress also delegated both executive and judicial-like oversight to HHS. The executive oversight operated primarily through the renewal of the contracts for administration of the OPTN and the SRTR but also through ex officio participation in meetings. The judicial-like oversight operates through the authority of the HHS secretary to make rules de jure. Although it does so less conventionally than regulatory agencies, the OPTN falls under what Rosenbloom called "tripartite custody," a characteristic of federal administration since passage of the Administrative Procedure Act in 1946 (2000, 150).

Conclusion

Assessing institutional performance poses both positive and normative problems. The positive problem stems from the fact that the outcomes that would have been produced by the counterfactual institution cannot be observed and the empirical basis for estimating them is thin. The normative problem is choosing the values, or goals, to be used to assess the outcomes. The positive assessment of the OPTN looked at the processes that produced rules in several areas, including the most important rules for kidney and liver allocation, and drew on our general knowledge of agency regulation to argue that the evolution of these rules would have been different had rulemaking been done by HHS. Specifically, I assert that rulemaking by the OPTN is more frequent, incremental, evidence-based, and open than HHS rulemaking would be. Without arguing for specific goals, it is not possible to make a definitive statement about whether the OPTN produces better policy than HHS would. However, as transplant technology and knowledge progress quickly, frequent rule changes seem to be a necessary condition for good policy. Combined with reliance on evidence and value consciousness, it may be enough. My overall assessment is that the OPTN produces better rules than HHS would through conventional rulemaking.

9

Is the OPTN a Viable and Desirable Model in other Medical Contexts?

Every form of governance has strengths and weaknesses. I believe that the account of the OPTN shows that it offers a favorable balance of strengths over weaknesses for setting and implementing organ transplantation policy. Most important, it is quite an effective arrangement for integrating expertise, values, and interests. It is exemplary in bringing evidence and tacit knowledge to rulemaking. It also is commendable in promoting the consideration of competing values, although the predominant process of incremental change from initially adopted rules tends to result in relatively slow responses to concerns that particular values are receiving too little weight. With the notable exception of the controversy over liver allocation during the promulgation of the Final Rule, it accommodates competing interests enough to keep stakeholders committed to participation in its deliberative processes. It can even produce nonincremental change, although rarely, as with more familiar forms of governance. Especially in comparison to conventional agency regulation, the private rulemaking of the OPTN seems to be desirable for organ transplantation. Does it, though, offer any lessons relevant to designing governance arrangements in other areas of medicine?

This chapter seeks to answer this question two ways. First, it reconsiders the OPTN from the perspective of institutional design. Specifically, it identifies key features that enable the OPTN to function effectively as a private rulemaker. Although it is unwise to assume that institutional features that function in particular ways ensemble will necessarily do so when used individually, identifying and characterizing them individually is certainly a first step in assessing their potential usefulness in other contexts.

Second, it considers possible applications of the design elements in two other medical contexts: governing electronic records to promote effective evidence-based learning, and, most boldly, using private rulemaking to improve the allocation of resources for surgery in the United States. Specifically, it considers how private rulemaking could be used to implement a global budget constraint on federal reimbursement for surgical services to encourage surgeries that are cost-effective, discourage those that are not, and promote developing and applying evidence for making these decisions.

The OPTN as Institutional Design

The governance of complex policy areas in representative democracies generally demands complex arrangements to achieve acceptable balance among technical efficiency, accountability, and economy. This generalization certainly applies to the OPTN. Yet recognizing that, in the context of institutional design, the whole is always more than the sum of the parts, it is nonetheless useful at least to identify key features that contribute to its effectiveness in producing continuous informed adjustments to policy aimed at furthering desirable goals. Eight features seem particularly important in the operation of the OPTN: professional engagement, continuity, meaningful stakes, decision making by voting, specialization with consultation, transparency, data for creating evidence, and strategic oversight.

Professional Engagement

Expertise and practice-related values distinguish professions. Professionals typically enjoy a high status that reflects the investments in knowledge and craft skills they must master and the commitment they make to particular values. Professional norms, which express these values in terms of the duties professionals owe to those they serve, typically arise through self-regulation but often become formalized in law. Engaging professionals in policymaking offers the potential not only for tapping their expertise but also for giving voice to their norms.

Doctors, nurses, epidemiologists, and other medical professionals have the essential substantive expertise needed for effective medical governance. They also share a background in science that gives them at least some familiarity with making inferences from empirical evidence. Engaging them in rulemaking not only taps their substantive expertise, but also brings to the table generally greater methodological sophistication than enjoyed by the general public or professions such as law. This does not eliminate disputes over inference, but it does provide a framework for focusing debate and identifying relevant questions that could be answered empirically. In other words, it facilitates an evidence-based approach.

The shared values these professionals bring to governance may also be important. The potential of professional norms as a resource in regulatory design has been noted by Eugene Bardach and Robert Kagan (1982). For example, appropriate professional norms for avoiding health risks could be engaged by requiring firms to have industrial hygienists with the authority to shut down production lines when threats to worker health arise. In the rulemaking context, there is at least the possibility that norms concerning the welfare of patients will temper self-interest.

Professionals may also bring legitimacy to the rulemaking process. To the extent that the public and their elected representatives trust professionals to pursue particular values consistent with social welfare, they may be more willing to defer to the professionals, making them authoritative in their domains of expertise. In the United States, physicians still enjoy considerable trust that contributes to their authority and political legitimacy.

The level of trust in the medical profession, however, appears to have eroded somewhat over the last fifty years (Schlesinger 2002). These declines are probably related to the changing nature of health care arrangements, such as the move from individual practice to managed care, that increase the perceived risk of trusting physicians (Mechanic 1998) and perhaps to the fragmentation of organized medicine, with physicians increasingly seeing the societies that represent their specialties as their primary representatives (Stevens 2001). Mark Schlesinger concludes that elites now seem less accepting of medical authority than the public and that "the erosion of medical authority in American politics can be attributed largely to concerns about medical efficacy, the failure of physicians to preserve their altruistic image treating the poor, and the lack of trust in the political involvement of the medical profession" (2002, 224). The influence of medical authority is now more likely to depend on the governance arrangements within which it is exercised.

Rulemaking by the OPTN relies heavily on the participation of transplant professionals who bring relevant expertise to the table. The norm of promoting patient welfare and a shared understanding of science help shape deliberations to be value-overt and evidence-based. The OPTN experience is more likely to be transferable to other areas of medical governance, where medical professionals would be important participants, than to other applications lacking a dominant profession with appropriate expertise and socially valued norms.

Continuity

Institutions can be defined as "relatively stable sets of widely shared and generally realized expectations about how people will behave in particular social, economic, and political circumstances" (Weimer 1997, 2). Thus, by definition, habituated behavior and continuity are the normal state of affairs for institutions. The OPTN is an institution by virtue of both its formally delegated authorities and the generally realized expectations about how it will exercise those authorities. Its internal organization and practices create and maintain these expectations. Specifically, standing committees with clear jurisdictions, multiyear memberships with staggered terms, and assigned support staff give continuity to policy development and implementation.

The continuity enables the committees to deal effectively with many inherently complicated issues by providing an opportunity for members to learn about them over their two-year terms. The opportunity to learn is most important for those who do not have expertise directly relevant to the issue at hand, but it is also important for enabling those who do have such expertise to relate it directly to problems with existing policies and proposed alternatives for addressing the problems. Learning about other committee members through mutual participation may also increase trust in the information they provide. When major changes in policy are being developed, often over an extended period, committees may be allowed to expand so that existing members with appropriate expertise can be reappointed as new members are added. The Kidney Transplantation Committee, for example, retained a number of members for second terms during the development of the kidney allocation system proposal. The UNOS staff assigned to support committees contribute to learning by providing extensive meeting materials, meeting minutes, information about deliberations in other committees, and guidance on organizational procedures for making policy changes.

The continuity also promotes cooperation. One of the important conceptual insights of contemporary social science is that repeated interaction can induce cooperation that would not be possible in a one-time interaction (Schotter 1981; Taylor 1982; Hardin 1982; Axelrod 1982). In game-theoretic terms, cooperation can be an equilibrium strategy for players in a repeated game even when it is not an equilibrium in the stage game being repeated. The practical implication is that continuity, both of the decision arena and of those within it, increases the chances that participants will acquiesce in the short run to adverse decisions in the expectation that they will be able to influence future decisions.

The nature of this continuous engagement with policy issues differs from that in conventional rulemaking. Although a regulatory agency may continuously assess policy in a particular area, only the most interested stakeholders are likely to communicate with it in the absence of a notice of proposed rulemaking. In the extreme, these most interested stakeholders "capture" the regulatory agency (Bernstein 1955) or, with the relevant congressional committees, form "iron triangles" that control policy (Lowi 1969), creating a continuity that favors their interests. Although these extremes have become rarer as the regulatory process has become more "conflictual, permeable, and unpredictable" (Gais, Peterson, and Walker 1984, 163), only the most interested stakeholders are likely to monitor and inform agencies during rule development. (Negotiated rulemaking seeks more comprehensive involvement of stakeholders during rule development, but only on a one-time basis.) Following a notice of proposed rulemaking, more stakeholders may volunteer information, but primarily in response to the rule rather than related to the nature of the problem, or other problems perhaps of more importance, or alternative rules.

The continuous involvement of stakeholders is most important when they have tacit knowledge relevant to the design of effective rules. Engaging a full range of stakeholders increases the chances that relevant information drawn from their tacit knowledge will be brought to the process. Engaging them as long-term participants may increase the likelihood of their being willing to reveal information that does not support the rules they prefer, especially because they may have to respond to problems that arise during implementation.

Meaningful Stakes

The time and energy of people with scarce expertise typically carries high opportunity costs. These experts, or their employers, are more likely to be willing to bear the costs of participating in governance when they perceive the stakes to be meaningful. For that to be the case, the stakes must involve something of value that can be influenced through the experts' participation in governance. Value often arises through scarcity, whether inherent or institutional. Goods like radio spectrum, cadaveric transplant organs, and airport landing slots have limited supplies, at least in the short run, that make them valuable and, therefore, their allocation meaningful. Rents created by agricultural cartels limiting supply make production quotas valuable and meaningful to growers. Hard budget constraints may make participation in spending decisions meaningful for those who can potentially benefit from allocations.

Even when what is at sake is important, participation in governance becomes more meaningful when it is consequential, connecting participation directly to outcomes. Clear delegations of authority to organizations to develop particular aspects of policy make participation in those organizations consequential. Relatively narrow and sharply circumscribed authorities are likely to be most consequential because they reduce the chances of competition with alternative authorities within the larger polity.

The OPTN has clear authority to develop policy concerning cadaveric organs, which have great value because they are the scarcest resource in organ transplantation. Although their availability can be affected by a variety of policies, such as those related to the determination of deceased-donor eligibility, the opportunities for live donations, and the incentives for transplant centers to expend effort in securing donations, their short-run supply is effectively fixed. Allocation rules are therefore consequential. Transplant surgeons and other highly skilled professionals contribute many hours to service on committees with reimbursement for travel and lodging expenses only. They are probably motivated to some extent by altruism and the benefits of professional association. The substantial commitments they make, however, almost certainly reflect their perceptions that the rules being made are particularly relevant to their ability to help their patients and realize the financial gains that flow from doing so.

The direct connection between expertise and policy in OPTN governance that makes the stakes for participants meaningful tends to be muted for regulatory advisory committees, for two reasons. First, advisory committees are often asked to separate science from policy and politics. Based on their comparative studies of federal advisory committees, Sheila Jasanoff (1990) and Bruce L. R. Smith (1992) conclude that committees are likely to be most effective when they do not limit their advice to questions of fact. Second, committee members rarely know the extent to which the advice they offer will influence agency decisions. The more tenuous the connection between their advice and policy, the less consequential they are likely to view their efforts.

Decision Making by Voting

Voting is an imperfect mechanism for aggregating individual preferences. Indeed, one of the few things we know with certainty in the social sciences is that voting cannot be perfected (Arrow 1951). Nonetheless, voting serves the very important instrumental purpose of allowing a decision to be made in the absence of consensus. In developing complex policies, voting may also be useful, at least temporarily, in specifying components needed to assemble a complete proposal and therefore move toward a final decision. Although voting can sometimes be sophisticated in the sense of people voting against their true preferences at the early stages of the process to obtain a more favorable final outcome, the proportions voting for and against a proposal generally convey information about the degree of consensus on the proposal.

The OPTN/UNOS board of directors approves policies and bylaws through majority rule voting. In addition, committees routinely vote on questions related to policies and bylaws. Particularly in developing complicated policy proposals, such as the kidney allocation score (KAS) proposal, these votes allow the process to move forward, resolving some issues so that attention can be focused on those that remain. Voting in committees also facilitates continuous incremental change to existing policies by enabling committees to achieve small wins, a series of concrete outcomes of moderate importance that may "attract allies, deter opponents, and lower resistance to subsequent proposals" (Weick 1984, 43). For example, the series of changes to liver allocation policy, including those that ensured the integrity of patient classification, contributed to the eventual introduction of the MELD/PELD system. More mundanely, the small wins may help keep committee members engaged by making them feel more effective.

Relying on majority rule voting may cause instability if the distribution of votes does not reflect the distribution of interests. In the case of the OPTN, the equal representation of small and large transplant centers gives the larger centers less influence than they would likely have in conventional regulation. This situation appears to have been in play with respect to liver allocation during the 1990s when the University of Pittsburgh Medical Center turned to the Department of Health and Human Services (HHS) after its efforts within the OPTN were frustrated.

Voting in the OPTN is unlike that in conventional regulation. Independent regulatory commissions take votes, but usually only on fully developed policy proposals—the actual development of the policy proposals, as with agency regulation, typically does not proceed through recorded votes. Regulatory agencies may engage advisory committees that record votes. However, as noted, these committees usually advise on scientific and technical matters, rather than policy development, and their votes thus rarely focus on specific policy choices.

Specialization with Consultation

Policy development often involves a tension between expertise and the full range of relevant values. Designing policies that can be effectively implemented in complex circumstances and predicting their consequences generally requires the tacit knowledge of specific experts. If these experts have similar experiences, they may also have similar values. It is therefore usually worthwhile to broaden the design process to include a wider range of knowledgeable participants, who may bring values to the process that might otherwise be ignored or only surface as controversy over the ultimately proposed policy.

In the case of the OPTN, the main locus of policy development is typically the standing committee with recognized jurisdiction. Most important, specific committees take primary responsibility for allocation of the various organs. These committees, which also include patient representatives and ex officio representatives of the SRTR and HHS, have a majority of members with substantial experience with that organ's transplantation, whether as surgeons or in another capacity. Policy changes usually emerge from these committees as proposals to the board of directors.

The organ committees consult regularly with other committees, including those with jurisdictions over general aspects of transplantation, such as patient affairs, minority affairs, and ethics. Consultation takes a number of forms, among them members of general committees serving as members of allocation committees, presentations to general committees by members of allocation committees, shared information and analyses, and requests to the general committees for comments on specific proposals. These mechanisms promote extensive consultation during policy development.

As with public rulemaking, the OPTN also seeks public comment on proposed policies after they have been developed. In both cases, the comments tend to come from the most interested stakeholders or from individuals mobilized by them. The responses are sometimes quite strong, particularly when groups of patients already on transplant waiting lists perceive policies as threatening their priorities. The board of directors may respond by rejecting the proposal or sending it back to the committees for redesign. For example, the proposal by several of the committees to begin waiting time accrual for kidney transplants at the onset of dialysis was rejected in the face of strong opposition from patients who had been listed either before or at the onset of dialysis. Interestingly, in many cases where policy changes were vocally opposed but nonetheless adopted, the controversy did not continue once implementation began.

Transparency

Some transparency in governance is a prerequisite for accountability and perhaps for legitimacy as well. National security concerns are often a rationale for limited transparency, despite the counterargument that in robust democracies transparency in fact promotes security (Roberts 2006, 42). Although in some circumstances there may be trade-offs between transparency and effective deliberation (Vermeule 2007), increasing the free flow of information about the processes and outcomes of governance is generally intrinsically desirable. Comparative analysis also suggests that it is instrumentally desirable. Countries with more accessible information about the economy and the government appear to govern better (Islam 2006). Greater transparency generally promotes better governance.

The OPTN deliberates about policy in public. With the exception of meetings to handle membership issues, anyone can attend committee meetings as observers. Although there is some variation by committee, meeting summaries and reports to the board of directors as well as executive summaries of the minutes of board meetings are routinely posted on the OPTN website. Those interested in participating in OPTN policy development can add their names to a list of people routinely sent requests for comments on proposed policies.

The SRTR is also very open in its fundamental tasks, including supporting OPTN policy development and providing researchers access to transplant data. It does not, however, provide ready electronic access on its own website to the analyses it produces for the OPTN. Most of these can be accessed only through OPTN committee reports. The most important analyses, though, often appear as chapters in the OPTN/SRTR *Annual Reports* published by HHS. Because the audience interested in analyses outside of their role in committee deliberations is probably very small, the lack of direct access through the

SRTR website has little relevance to meaningful transparency in the development of organ transplantation policy.

The transparency of OPTN governance prevents stakeholders from being surprised by policy decisions. The deliberative process provides many avenues for involvement in policy development—participation in committees, contact with committee members, and comments on proposed policies. At times, stakeholders have mobilized potentially interested parties, such as patients with a particular disease or organizations with missions related to specific diseases, to send comments. The board of directors is thus rarely surprised by reactions to policies. Especially because policies can have life and death implications for patients on transplant waiting lists, transparent deliberations during policy development almost certainly add to the legitimacy of the policies that result, perhaps at the cost of greater difficulty in making nonincremental changes.

The transparency of policy development within the OPTN contrasts with the largely opaque process of policy development through conventional rulemaking (West 2005). The primary source of information on rule developments under way is the Semiannual Regulatory Agenda (Unified Agenda), which has been assembled and published by the Office of the Federal Register since 1983 and made available electronically since 1994. Until 2007, when the criteria for listing were narrowed to focus on rules with significant economic impact on a large number of small entities, agencies were required to list all the proposed and final regulations they expected to issue in the upcoming year. Monitoring the Unified Agenda allows interested parties to communicate with the agency during rule development. Indeed, Susan Webb Yackee finds evidence that interested parties do engage in influential ex parte communications with the agencies, but that this process favors resource-rich interests (2008). However, as the title of Yackee's paper— "The Hidden Politics of Regulation"—makes clear, the rule development process is far from transparent. Indeed, only in the case of negotiated rulemaking, which directly involves stakeholders in rule development, is the process nearly as transparent as it is within the OPTN.

In theory, the notice and comment requirements of the Administrative Procedure Act give transparency to the process through which proposed rules are finalized. Comments are accumulated in a docket open to public inspection and the final rulemaking must address them. However, until fairly recently, inspection of the docket usually required an interested party to visit a particular office in the Washington, DC, area in person, an expense likely to be reasonable only for those with the largest stakes. The E-Government Act of 2002 (Public Law 107-347) sought to reduce these costs by requiring agencies to move toward electronic dockets that would reduce the costs of submitting and inspecting comments. Although some scholars predicted that the move to electronic access would greatly increase public participation in rulemaking (Johnson 1998), an analysis of the impact of the introduction of the electronic docket by the Department of Transportation before the act found no change in patterns of participation (Balla and Daniels 2007). If one believes that collective decisions about the allocation of medical services should be transparent, then additional mechanisms should be developed to open up conventional regulation even further to potentially interested parties.

Data for Creating Evidence

In the 1990s evidence-based medicine arose as the "most important contemporary initiative committed to reshaping biomedical reason and practice" (Mykhalovskiy and Weir 2004, 1059). It can be defined as "the conscientious, explicit, and judicious use of current best evidence in making decisions about the care of individual patients. The practice of evidence-based medicine means integrating individual clinical expertise with the best available external clinical evidence from systematic research" (Sackett et al. 1996, 71).

Systematic research to assess the effectiveness of medical interventions requires data linking the interventions to meaningful outcomes. Data generated by true experiments, with random assignment of patients into treatment and control groups, enjoy a privileged position among researchers. If generated through well-designed and well-executed experiments, such data offer a high degree of internal validity in terms of assessing the treatment effects, especially in establishing causality. However, relying solely on experiments as a source of data would be a mistake for a number of reasons. First, experiments are generally costly and thus not widely undertaken, and when they are undertaken, budget constraints tend to limit total sample sizes so that only a small number of treatments can be assessed. Second, ethical issues often arise in denying the expected better treatment to those in the control group or in subjecting those in the treatment group to treatments with unknown risks. Third, the high costs of maintaining experimental integrity over extended periods tends to limit their use in assessing long-term effects. Fourth, because compliance with experimental protocols cannot always be maintained, differences often arise between the estimation of effects based on intent-to-treat analyses, which use all subjects initially assigned to groups whether or not they complied with the protocol for the group, and as-treated analyses, which attempt to relate outcomes to actual levels of compliance with group protocols. The former can guard against biases introduced by such confounding effects as sicker patients dropping out or crossing over to other groups, but they may not provide an appropriate prediction of the treatment effects that would result in clinical situations where compliance is achieved.

Data generated through, or as a by-product of, clinical practice is almost always inferior to data from well-planned and well-executed experiments that guard against self-selection or steering into treatment modalities. Nonetheless, clinical data can still be of great value, especially if they comprehensively cover relevant groups of patients and include high quality measures of outcomes. Clinical data may provide the only practical way to gather large enough samples to find rare but significant effects or to find effects that manifest only after long periods.

The SRTR is an exemplary clinical database. It includes a near universe of transplant candidates and it follows transplant recipients over an extended period. The OPTN contributes to the quality and appropriateness of the data in the registry through the policies it sets concerning reporting by transplant centers. Analyses using the data, primarily statistical and simulation models developed by SRTR staff, play an important role in policy development and evaluation efforts of the OPTN committees: it provides systematic evidence to complement the tacit knowledge of their members. Arguably, because of the registry data and its use by the SRTR and the OPTN, organ transplantation is at the forefront of evidence-based medicine.

The availability of data to produce relevant evidence during policy development is especially important in the face of conflicting values and sometimes divergent interests. Balancing important values, such as fairness and efficiency, is difficult in the abstract. An empirical basis for understanding the possible trade-offs between them creates a more manageable choice problem. This was certainly the case in the development of the KAS proposal, where its final version reflected a series of revisions to increase fairness at the loss of some net benefit.

Empirical analysis also allows investigation of the various claims put forward in support of positions. For example, the models of liver allocation used during the Final Rule controversy showed relatively small gains, if any, from national rather than local priority in allocation. Absent data to create relevant evidence, one might wonder whether the OPTN committees would be able to achieve enough agreement to continue to engage effectively in continuous policy revision.

Strategic Oversight

Delegation of authority within representative government demands some sort of oversight to guide and monitor those exercising the authority. The most familiar delegations flow from legislatures to public agencies. Legislatures oversee agencies in a variety of ways, from routine monitoring, so-called police patrol, to event-triggered or interest group prompted scrutiny, so-called fire alarms (McCubbins and Schwartz 1984). Public agencies also often delegate, either by choice or by mandate, to other entities, including other levels of government and private organizations. In these delegations, the agencies provide the primary oversight. Effective governance requires that oversight be appropriate for the delegation. Of course, it should be strategic in the sense of anticipating the reactions of the overseen, but it should also be strategic in the sense of promoting broad social goals rather than prescribing specific policies.

Congress created the OPTN as a distinct entity but made it subject to HHS oversight. The oversight role with respect to organ procurement and allocation policies was initially ambiguous. The initial follow-up legislation seemed to strengthen the independence of the OPTN. Nonetheless, HHS asserted its authority over making OPTN rules binding, establishing a distinction between de jure rules that have the force of law and de facto rules that actually govern transplantation.

Aside from accepting, rejecting, or requiring OPTN actions through rulemaking, HHS exercises oversight in managing the contracts to administer the OPTN and the SRTR. Although each has a legislative basis, and the OPTN effectively has its own taxing power in setting fees for placing patients on waiting lists, HHS selects the organizations that administer them. Initially, both were administered by UNOS, the administrator of the voluntary network of transplant centers that predated the creation of the OPTN. Later HHS took the contract for SRTR away from UNOS, establishing the current arrangement of separate administrators. The ex officio membership of HHS personnel on OPTN committees facilitates ongoing monitoring of policy development and implementation. These memberships reciprocally provide committees with information about what to expect from the otherwise largely opaque processes operating within HHS.

Since the resolution of the Final Rule controversy, HHS has engaged in what might be termed strategic oversight—sparing and selective interventions to guide or direct the OPTN and SRTR. The Final Rule that ultimately emerged requires review of allocation rules in terms of general goals, but does not specify how those goals are to be met. Most important, HHS has not attempted to formalize or overturn any of the OPTN substantive allocation rules, but rather allows them to operate de facto. By contrast, it has acted to make OPTN rules on data reporting by transplant centers and organ procurement organizations legally binding so that OPTN efforts to ensure compliance have the force of law. The HHS has also been strategic in directing the SRTR to develop new simulation models for assessing changes in organ allocation policies.

These selective and facilitating interventions contrast with the blunt effort during the Final Rule controversy to push the OPTN toward sharing livers and other organs nationally. That effort was rebuffed politically by a congressional moratorium and largely scientifically by the Institute of Medicine study mandated by Congress. It elicited court challenges and played out over a number of years before the less intrusive version of the Final Rule ultimately emerged. Although the controversy was extraordinary in many respects, it nonetheless gives a sobering view of how contentious organ allocation policy making could be if it were to be routinely set through conventional rulemaking. The possibility of overturning or preempting OPTN policies, or even replacing the OPTN contractor, gives HHS considerable leverage. However, because these actions would likely have costly consequences for all parties, they are most effective when they remain threats rather than actions. In game theoretic terms, they constitute a punishment path that helps keep HHS and the OPTN on an equilibrium path of cooperation.

Private Rulemaking in other Medical Contexts

The appropriateness of governance arrangements depends on the context in which they will operate. As argued in chapter 2, private rulemaking, like that by the OPTN, is likely to be technically efficient when the stakeholders have the necessary expertise and changing circumstances, such as an accumulation of evidence relevant to good practice, require frequent adjustment of rules. Private rulemaking is most likely to be politically attractive when it allows legislators, or public executives, to avoid situations in which they face an unfavorable credit claiming and blame avoidance calculus and it can be based on an existing model of stakeholder cooperation. Although a history of cooperation among stakeholders is the most relevant model, the detailed assessment of the OPTN provides at least a generic model for thinking about governance design.

The design of governance incorporating private rulemaking should reflect those features identified as conducive to the effectiveness of the OPTN. The starting point almost certainly has to be the creation of meaningful stakes. This can be done in a number of ways. A narrow but clear delegation of authority is one approach, either as an explicit delegation of rulemaking authority, as in determining the content of the Vaccines for Children Program by the Advisory Committee on Immunization Practices, or a delegation of agenda setting authority, as in ranking diagnosis-treatment pairs by the Oregon Health Services Commission. Another approach is to couple allocation authority with induced scarcity by imposing a hard budget constraint, in effect following the advice of Alice Rivlin for dealing the professionalized areas like medicine: "Put the money on the stump and run" (1983, 6). The two applications that follow use these approaches.

Interoperable Medical Records

The routine use of electronic medical records offers potential administrative savings and reductions in medical errors. If the records are interoperable, they provide a network externality by allowing more seamless movement of information about patients among health care providers. These are the benefits that accrue directly to patients, providers, and third-party payers. Health services researchers have also recognized the public good nature of universal electronic medical records in terms of supporting evidence-based medicine (Olsen, Aisner, and McGinnis 2007, 5–6). Some see databases of electronic health records as filling important knowledge gaps in evidence-based medicine and promoting a "rapid-learning" health care system (Etheredge 2007). Nonetheless, despite the widespread calls for effective electronic medical records for the past thirty years, their adoption has been slow. For example, a survey conducted in 2002 found that systems that allow doctors and other health professionals to issue medical orders, such as for medications, were available in less than 10 percent of U.S. hospitals (Ash et al. 2004).

A number of obstacles stand in the way of interoperability, especially semantic interoperability, which allows the exchange of information in defined terms and expressions (Hoffman and Podgurski 2008). The medical lexicon is itself complicated, with variation in meanings and abbreviations across specialties and regions. Vendors have already invested in proprietary formats and data structures that cannot directly communicate. Sharona Hoffman and Andy Podgurski note the potential financial disincentives for interoperability (2008). Most obviously, vendors would no longer enjoy a lock-in effect with current customers and thus would be subject to greater competition. Providers and clinicians may fear that the ability to move medical records easily would increase patient mobility. Clinicians may also fear that more effective ownership of the records by patients would open them up to greater monitoring and potentially greater malpractice liability. Although there have been some successful voluntary initiatives to increase interoperability, such as efforts to facilitate standards for exchange of information among hospital information systems over the last two decades, it is unlikely that meaningful interoperability will be achieved without some government involvement.

In 2004 President Bush issued Executive Order 13335, which established within HHS the position of national health information technology coordinator, charged with promoting "nationwide interoperable health information infrastructure" in collaboration with relevant executive agencies and "private parties of interest, including consumers, providers, payers, and administrators." The HHS secretary established an advisory committee, the American Health Information Community (AHIC), to make recommendations concerning an interoperability framework and to provide a forum for participation by stakeholders. Its charter also called for it to make recommendations concerning the establishment of a private sector organization that would succeed it.

In August 2007 HHS issued a white paper that set out a vision for a successor to the AHIC (HHS 2007a). Membership in AHIC 2.0, as it was known, would be open to the entire health community, which would be organized into sectors, such as clinicians, consumers, and government. It suggested the possibility of a distinction between direct members, who would have voting rights and pay fees, and participating members, typically individuals affiliated with direct members, who would neither pay fees nor have voting rights. The governing body would be a board of directors providing balanced representation for the various sectors. The actual development would be done by a grantee. At a public hearing on the proposal, HHS Secretary Michael Leavitt offered a rationale for structuring AHIC 2.0 as a public-private partnership:

> When it comes down to it, there [are] only three ways to set standards. First, you can have government set them, and we'll probably get them wrong because we'll do it in a vacuum. Or second, you can use what I call the "last vendor standing," which is just to wait to see who eliminates who, but that doesn't work in this space because we've found several different ways you can accomplish the same goal. Or third, you can go through this kind of process, and it's hard, and it's painful, and it's slow, but nevertheless, when you get there you have something everybody's agreed upon. Once that's occurred, the government needs to utilize its regulatory functions in a way that supports those standards, as opposed to dictating those standards. (Leavitt 2007, 14)

The white paper and Leavitt's comments suggest that AHIC 2.0 would be like a private standard setter whose standards gain force through conventional regulatory action. Those involved with the development of AHIC 2.0 point to standard-setting organizations, such as the American National Standards Institute, the National Quality Forum, and the North American Energy Standards Board, as possible models.

A grant for organizing and launching AHIC 2.0 was awarded to two nonprofit organizations, LMI Government Consulting and the Brookings Institution. By July 2008 the LMI-Brookings team incorporated the AHIC successor and began a process to select the initial twenty-one members of its board of directors. The new board will specify the nuts and bolts of the organization, ranging from membership criteria and representation of membership within the board to funding.

One can imagine a variety of governance designs emerging, including ones that would be closer to private rulemaking than private standard setting. There would likely be meaningful stakes for most medical information system vendors even if the AHIC successor set standards that required affirmative HHS action to become effective. These stakes could be amplified by a general HHS rule that medical information systems purchased with funds from federal sources be provided by vendors who were members of AHIC 2.0. By making compliance with the adopted standards a condition of membership, the standards would become de facto rules without formal HHS action. Based on the OPTN experience, one would predict that this arrangement would facilitate continuous incremental development of the set of rules governing interoperability. De facto rules that proved impractical or undesirable in practice could more easily be modified than if they were established de jure by HHS.

Inducing vendor participation through a membership requirement for selling systems to entities using federal funds would make it possible to finance AHIC 2.0 through fees based on the number of patients covered by each vendor's systems—analogous to those for putting patients on the transplant waiting lists that provide most of the funding for the OPTN. The rates could be set to cover AHIC 2.0 administrative costs. Reimbursing members for travel and lodging expenses incurred in committee work and that of other AHIC 2.0 activities could help expand the set of stakeholders who would be active members. Participation would also be facilitated by maximum transparency, including fully open committee meetings and conscientious posting of agendas and minutes on the AHIC Successor website.

One can imagine the value of a companion organization that would play a role similar to that of the SRTR in supporting the OPTN. For purposes of discussion, imagine that HHS provided contract support to an organization to operate what would be called the National Archive for Medical Electronic Records (NAMER). The contractor would be responsible for assembling data from medical records, assessing and reporting the quality of these data to the AHIC successor, and preparing analytical data sets of de-identified data and making them available to researchers. The narrow purpose of these activities would be to help AHIC 2.0 assess the effectiveness of its efforts. Their broader purpose would be to ensure that AHIC 2.0 standards facilitate realization of the public good—general medical knowledge—that interoperable medical records potentially offer.

The NAMER would contribute to these goals through its efforts to convert medical records to analytical data sets. During this process, relevant weaknesses would be identified so that they could be addressed in standards. The quality of what is collected, in terms of both accuracy and completeness, is obviously important for research and probably for clinical practice as well. In some cases, however, there may be some data items that are not relevant to clinical practice but that would be valuable for research. For example, closing records with dates and causes of death are not directly relevant to treatment of the patient but could be very valuable in assessing treatments given before death.

In terms of moving toward the rapid-learning health system, the NAMER would overcome some of the barriers that researchers face in making full use of the available electronic records. Most important, the NAMER could help researchers meet patient confidentiality requirements imposed by the Health Insurance Portability and Accountability Act (Public Law 104-191) by linking medical records needed for research and supplying the data to researchers without patient identification. Fees would be charged to researchers, who would include them in their peer-reviewed grant proposals, to cover the marginal costs of assembling the data sets. As the use of electronic records spread, and experience in making the data useful for research accumulated, the capacity for evidence-based medicine would increase.

Making the AHIC successor a private rulemaker would require relatively modest changes in the arrangements that appear to be taking shape. As such, it does not shed light on how the OPTN model might be used as the basis for a truly novel approach in some areas of medical governance. The next section considers how the OPTN model could be used to promote evidence-based practice and cost-effectiveness with respect to surgery.

Replication of the OPTN Model: A Medicare Surgery Budget

In the United States, surgeries are numerous, expensive, and often lack solid evidence regarding their efficacy or cost-effectiveness. In 2006 there were more than 32 million surgeries performed in U.S. short-stay hospitals on an inpatient basis, including more than 10 million for the primary Medicare population, those sixty-five and older (DeFrances et al. 2007, 16). Although statistics are not as systematically collected on outpatient or ambulatory surgeries, an analysis of data from seventeen states on surgeries performed in 2003 found roughly equal numbers of outpatient and inpatient surgeries (Russo et al. 2007, table 1); the proportion of outpatient surgeries now appears to be more than 60 percent (National Center for Health Statistics 2007, 352). The inpatient prospective payment system used by Medicare Part A reimburses hospitals for nonphysician surgical costs according to diagnosis related groups (DRGs) that depend on the surgical procedures used. In 2005 the physician services payment system used by Medicare Part B paid about $58 billion to physicians for their medical services, including more than $8.5 billion to thirteen surgical specialties (HHS 2008). With Medicare Part A spending roughly two dollars for in-patient hospital services for each Part B dollar, the total Medicare costs of surgery would have been about $25 billion annually. With a ratio of 4:1 for total surgeries to surgeries for those sixty-five and older, and Medicare reimbursing at roughly 80 percent of the private rate, the total surgical bill in the United States in 2005 was probably about $120 billion.

Assessing the appropriateness of the large annual expenditures on surgeries requires knowledge about the efficacy and cost-effectiveness of the various types of surgeries in the contexts in which they are used. Unlike new pharmaceuticals, which are regulated by the Food and Drug Administration, surgical procedures do not require well-controlled studies to demonstrate their effectiveness and safety before they enter mainstream practice. As Alan Gerber and Eric Patashnik note in their account of arthroscopic surgery to treat osteoarthritis of the knee, at least since the 1970s, medical critics have recognized the weak evidentiary basis typically advanced in support of new surgical procedures (2006). Gerber and Patashnik point out the lack of research on the effectiveness of even widely adopted surgical procedures as well as failure of the surgical professions and the Medicare program to make use of the evidence that is available.

A recent study of angioplasty illustrates the problem of the failure to follow established guidelines for surgery (Lin et al. 2008). Percutaneous coronary intervention, commonly referred to as angioplasty, is commonly used to treat coronary artery disease. It appears, however, to be no more effective in terms of death or myocardial infarction than less expensive treatments involving drugs and life-style changes. Because studies have shown that its use in patients with minimal symptoms appears on average to produce adverse outcomes, guidelines jointly issued by three relevant medical societies recommend that moderate or severe ischemia in stable angina patients be documented through noninvasive tests, primarily stress tests, before proceeding with angioplasty. Grace Lin and her colleagues found that only about 45 percent of stable patients with Medicare fee-for-service coverage had stress tests within ninety days before their angioplasties (2008). In other words, it appears that a majority of procedures were performed in contradiction to evidence-based guidelines. George Diamond and Sanjay Kaul note that one reason for the underuse of stress tests before angioplasty may be that the guidelines are not clear (2008). Nonetheless, they recommend that Medicare payments for angioplasties performed on stable patients without stress tests be reimbursed at a lower rate than those performed following stress tests that document the moderate to severe ischemia called for in the guidelines.

The differential payment proposal applies the strategy of fee-for-benefit rather than fee-for-services (Denton and Diamond 1995). In view of its failure to follow up on the findings of the controlled trial of arthroscopic knee surgery (Gerber and Patashnik 2006), however, it does not seem likely that the Centers for Medicare and Medicaid Services (CMS) would take steps on its own to implement the fee-for-benefit strategy. More generally, despite the increasing efforts of the CMS, the Agency for Healthcare Research and Quality, the National Institutes of Health, and the Department of Veterans Affairs to generate information on the comparative effectiveness of medical and surgical interventions, the Medicare Payment Advisory Commission (MedPAC) has concluded that there is currently not enough credible "information available to patients, providers, and payers to make informed treatment decisions" (Miller 2007, 1). MedPAC went on to raise several possibilities for creating a more effective governance arrangement to support the generation and assessment of information on comparative effectiveness, including a public-private entity, like the Federal Reserve, or a purely private entity. The purpose of this exercise is to sketch briefly how an entity modeled after the OPTN could play this role for surgery, perhaps providing a mechanism for heeding the call of Miriam Laugesen for "greater direct responsibility by physicians for higher quality and medically effective services and greater oversight of what Medicare pays for, perhaps informed by comparative effectiveness" (2009, 176). For ease of reference, this entity is called the Medicare Surgery Assessment Volunteers for Effectiveness (MedSAVE).

Like the OPTN, MedSAVE would be created through legislation. Its primary function would be to assess the effectiveness and cost-effectiveness of surgeries. The stakes would be made meaningful for participants by combining an overall annual budget for surgical services paid through Medicare Part B with the authority to set payment rates for specific surgical services through majority voting by a board of directors. Membership would be open to organizations representing surgeons and the surgical specialties, other organizations representing those concerned about specific diseases and the elderly, medical ethicists, and interested individuals drawn from the general public, patients, and the professions. Funding would be provided to support a full-time staff, a companion registry of surgeries like the SRTR, and participation expenses for individual members through a small surtax on surgeries paid for by Medicare. Table 9–1 summarizes MedSAVE in terms of the design features identified as contributing to the effectiveness of the OPTN.

Participants and general governance structure.   The OPTN formalized the existing voluntary network for organ sharing. Are there any existing institutional arrangements upon which MedSAVE could be built?

One possibility is to incorporate it within the Medicare Payment Advisory Commission, which, as discussed in chapter 2, plays an important role in advising Congress and HHS. However, doing so might jeopardize its larger mission of offering independent advice about the entire Medicare program. Another possibility would be to build on the Medicare Evidence Development and Coverage Advisory Committee (MEDCAC), which CMS uses to help it assess the evidence relevant to various clinical topics. Originally established in 1998 as the Medicare Coverage Advisory Committee, MEDCAC has up to eighty-eight at-

Table 9–1   OPTN Design Elements in MedSAVE

Professional engagement	Participation of surgeons with conflicting interests but with relevant expertise and some shared norms
Continuity	Legislative creation with dedicated funding source to create expectation of permanence; professional staff to support efforts of board of directors and committees
Meaningful stakes	Determination of Medicare fee schedule for surgeries subject to hard budget constraint with across-the-board fee reductions as default
Decision making by voting	Board of directors votes on fee schedule and data reporting requirements; committees vote on recommendations to the board of directors
Specialization with consultation	Majority of members scientific or clinical experts; committees focus on both categories of surgery and crosscutting issues
Transparency	Meetings of the board of directors and committees open to public; web posting of minutes and supporting studies
Data for creating evidence	Data reporting requirements set by board of directors to help assess surgical efficacy; collection, refinement, and analysis of data by SRTR-like unit
Strategic oversight	CMS appoints nonsurgical members to board of directors and has ex officio representation on the board of directors and committees

Source: Author's compilation.

large members, including up to six patient representatives, with voting rights. In addition, it includes up to six consumer representatives and up to six industry representatives. Calls for nominations are made in the *Federal Register* and stakeholders may submit nominations directly to CMS.

Subsets of the members of MEDCAC convene several times per year in public meetings to address specific questions posed by CMS. After reviewing available evidence and hearing testimony presented by interested parties, the committee members "vote" on the questions using various formats, such as five-point scales from low to high, or not likely to very likely. Average scores are reported for both voting and all participating members. For example, a meeting that dealt with spinal fusion for the treatment of low back pain took votes on the following question: "What level of confidence does the evidence provide in addressing the outcomes needed to determine the effectiveness of lumbar spinal fusion for low back pain due to lumbar degenerative disc disease?" The average score on a 5-point scale was 2.89 for nine voting members and 3.00 for the fourteen members overall (HHS 2006b, 12). These scores were advisory to CMS.

MEDCAC's purely advisory role limits its usefulness as a model for MedSAVE. Nonetheless, it indicates the sort of people with general expertise who would be sought out to participate in MedSAVE. MedSAVE would require explicit and systematic representation of the surgical specialties, however. The board of directors, which would have responsibility for approving surgical payment schedules, would be broadly representative but also include representatives selected by the American College of Surgeons, the American Academy of Ophthalmology, the American Academy of Orthopaedic Surgeons, the American Academy of Otolaryngology, the American Association of Neurological Surgeons, the American College of Obstetricians and Gynecologists, the American Pediatric Surgical Association, the American Society of Colon and Rectal Surgeons, the American Society of Plastic Surgeons, the American Urological Association, the Society for Vascular Surgery, and the Society of Thoracic Surgeons. Other organizations representing the medical professions, those interested in specific diseases, the elderly, and taxpayers would be invited to nominate people to participate in MedSAVE committees and the board of directors. So, for example, the board of directors might consist of the representatives appointed by the surgical societies and an equal number of people selected by CMS to represent broader medical and societal interests.

MedSAVE would create standing committees to advise the board of directors with recorded votes. Some of these committees would likely focus on specific surgical specializations and others would address crosscutting issues, such as standards for evidence, ethical concerns, and the development of coherent fee schedule proposals. A professional staff, funded from the surgery surtax, would support the work of the committees and the board of directors. The surtax would also provide funds for a sister organization, like the SRTR, that would assemble relevant data on surgical effectiveness, analyze it as requested by the MedSAVE committees, and make it available to researchers generally.

Health and Human Services would exercise strategic oversight in several ways. First, CMS would appoint the nonsurgical specialists to the board of directors. Second, CMS would have ex officio representation on the board of directors and the committees, and it would be responsible for ensuring that decision making within MedSAVE remained transparent. Third, the secretary of HHS would have the option of overruling the fee schedule adopted by MedSAVE and forcing across-the-board reductions. This last form of oversight employs what Bradley Karkkainen calls a "regulatory penalty default," a provision that imposes harsh terms on regulated parties who fail to produce acceptable alternatives voluntarily (2006, 869). It would be the sword on the wall that could be used if MedSAVE failed to carry out its responsibility to promote efficacy and efficiency in the provision of surgery to Medicare patients.

Money on the stump: The surgical budget constraint. Health care systems around the world have used four types of targets to control costs: price, volume, capacity, and appropriateness (White 1999). MedSAVE would use three of these. A combination of price and volume targets would set a global maximum on expenditures for surgical services similar to the one currently used for all physician services under Medicare Part B, and the members of MedSAVE would have an incentive to assess the appropriateness of types and circumstances of surgeries and discourage inappropriate surgeries through the fee schedule.

Originally, Medicare reimbursed physicians at rates that were "customary, prevailing, and reasonable." The Social Security Amendments of 1972 (Public Law 92-603) sought to slow the growth in Medicare expenditures by limiting the rate of increase in the fees paid for physician services to an index based on the average increase in physicians' costs of doing business. However, expenditures continued to grow rapidly as physicians increased the volume of services they provided to Medicare patients. The Omnibus Budget Reconciliation Act of 1989 (Public Law 101-239) authorized setting fee schedules for physicians providing services to Medicare beneficiaries based primarily on physician time, skill, intensity, practice expenses, malpractice insurance costs, and geographic area. It also imposed volume standards, limits on the growth in the number of procedures, intended to control the annual increase in expenditures. The fee schedules, which went into effect in 1992, were accompanied by annual volume standards for surgical, primary care, and nonsurgical services that sought to limit the increase in total expenditures for Medicare Part B.

The Balanced Budget Act of 1997 (Public Law 105-33) replaced the volume standards with the sustainable growth rate (SGR) system, which set both annual and cumulative targets for Medicare Part B spending. The SGR itself depends on several factors. the esti mated percentage change in physician fees, the estimated percentage change in the number of fee-for-service Medicare beneficiaries, the estimated percentage growth in real gross domestic product per capita (ten-year moving average), and the estimated percentage changes resulting from changes in laws and regulations. Beginning in 2002, the SGR target required across-the-board reductions in physician fees. The reduction called for in 2002, 5.4 percent, was actually implemented. However, in each of the following five years Congress intervened to block the implementation of reductions, instead allowing small increases in total expenditures to occur. As annual reductions for a number of years would be necessary to return actual expenditures to the SGR targets, it is quite likely that Congress will eventually modify the system.

Why has the SGR system been ineffective in controlling expenditure growth? As Rick Mayes and Robert Berenson note in their review of the Medicare prospective payment system, under the SGR "prudent physicians are penalized financially, while profligate ones are rewarded" because, from the perspective of the individual physician, gains from over-provision of services are larger than losses from contributions of those services to the overall fee reduction (2006, 92). Of course, this is just a tragedy of the commons, a classic common property resource problem in which individuals base their decisions on their private marginal benefits and costs, ignoring the contribution of their decisions to the average costs to all users of the resource. The most familiar approaches for countering such overconsumption are regulation and self-governance. With respect to the Medicare expenditure problem, regulation involves CMS taking steps to limit service use, which have been largely ineffective and often elicit opposition from the medical profession. Self-regulation involves the resource users, physicians receiving Medicare payments, taking actions to limit their collective overuse.

MedSAVE would provide the governance arrangements in which at least the surgical professions would have an incentive to self-regulate. The primary incentive would be the imposition of a separate SGR for surgeries, which would be implemented by calculating current total payments for surgeries under Medicare Part B as the starting point. In subsequent years the SGR would be used to calculate the new expenditure targets. Actual expenditures in excess of the target amount would trigger proportional reductions of all surgical payments in the subsequent year. MedSAVE, however, would have the authority to adjust the resource-based payments for surgeries so as to discourage inappropriate surgeries and reduce actual expenditures. The threat of across-the-board reductions in surgical fees, and the opportunity to influence the determination of inappropriate surgeries would provide the meaningful stakes to encourage participation in MedSAVE by the most relevant stakeholders, the surgical specialties.

Authorities: Payment rates and data requirements. The primary authority of MedSAVE would be to apply downward reductions to the resource-based fee schedule for surgeries currently in the Medicare Part B prospective payment system, what one can think of, for purposes of discussion, as full payment. MedSAVE could reduce the full payment to signal uncertainty about the effectiveness of a surgical procedure, or reduce it to zero to remove it from Medicare coverage entirely. MedSAVE would also have the authority to specify the conditions necessary for full payment. For example, returning to the angioplasty example, MedSAVE could specify that the full payment would be made in the case of stable angina patients only if moderate or severe ischemia is documented through a stress test before the procedure.

MedSAVE would also have the authority to require that specific data be collected before and after surgery as a condition of full payment. This authority could be used to produce data to provide better assessments of the effectiveness and safety of surgical procedures. Data requirements could be particularly useful in assessing both commonly used procedures of questionable effectiveness and new procedures.

Finally, MedSAVE would have the authority to use some of the financial resources it receives from the surtax on surgeries to fund research on surgical procedures. This research could include controlled experiments, perhaps using sham surgery methods where ethically appropriate, as well as observational studies based on administrative and required data. These studies would create evidence to support decision making by MedSAVE.

Potential benefits (and risks) of MedSAVE. If MedSAVE functioned as well as the OPTN, then the benefits could be substantial. Most important, MedSAVE would provide a framework for implementing evidence-based surgery by tapping the tacit knowledge of surgeons and creating incentives to develop data necessary to produce evidence about effectiveness. The driving force would be the opportunity to apply the scalpel to cut out inappropriate surgeries to avoid having the hatchet applied to fees across the board. MedSAVE would thus offer the potential of controlling the growth in a substantial component of Medicare Part B spending.

A successful MedSAVE would likely produce a number of desirable spillover effects. Reductions in unnecessary, ineffective, and dangerous surgeries would reduce hospitalization costs covered by Medicare Part A as well as physician costs. Many private insurers would take advantage of the signals sent by MedSAVE fee schedule adjustments in setting their own reimbursement rates and coverage. MedSAVE would become a model for efforts to tie the search for appropriate medical practice to expenditures controls in other categories of physician services.

Adopting MedSAVE would not be without risks. The OPTN formalized an existing network of a community of transplant surgeons that had experience voluntarily sharing organs among their transplant centers. MedSAVE would be a much more dramatic move. It would require cooperation across heterogeneous surgical specialties rather than within a single surgical community. The Final Rule controversy that engulfed the OPTN shows the potential vulnerability that MedSAVE would face if it failed to accommodate powerful surgical specializations that could attempt to overturn unfavorable decisions with appeals to HHS or Congress.

Perhaps the most relevant difference between MedSAVE and the OPTN is the scarcity that creates the high stakes. MedSAVE would require a budget constraint that, unlike the natural constraint of a limited number of cadaveric organs, is legislatively created and therefore subject to legislative change. Can Congress credibly commit to a fixed budget for surgery or for any other set of medical services for which we seek to induce evidence-based assessment? If not, the various interests might invest in lobbying Congress rather than in evidence-based medicine. Rather than conflicting with the promotion of good medical practice, more stringent cost control may actually be a prerequisite for more effective evidence-based medicine.

Failure of MedSAVE would involve loss of the resources invested in its creation and, perhaps more importantly, a setback for evidence-based medicine. Yet all medicine involves weighing benefits and risks. To realize the potential benefits of new forms of medical governance, taking some risk is necessary.

Conclusion

The empirical focus of this book is the OPTN, an unusual institution of medical governance that delegates the design of important rules to stakeholders. In view of the direct relevance of these rules to the lives and deaths of tens of thousands of Americans, simply understanding the operation of OPTN is a worthy enterprise for policy researchers. My ambition for this project, however, is to answer a more general question. What lessons can be drawn from the OPTN in designing governance arrangements in other medical contexts?

The first part of the answer involves a relatively familiar approach for social scientists. Drawing on the case at hand and the general findings of relevant research, a number of features appear to have contributed to the desirable outcomes observed. These features serve as a checklist against which alternative governance arrangements can be assessed. However, there is no guarantee that incorporating any proper subset of the features into a new institution would produce desirable results. As social scientists, we face the problem that we have too few comparable applications involving these features to allow us to determine which, if any, are either necessary or ample. As policy analysts seeking to deal with immediate problems, we cannot wait for serendipitous events to give us a better empirical basis for confident comparison of governance alternatives. Further, as policy analysts, we are forced to make predictions about what would happen if an alternative were adopted, rather than test hypotheses based on what has already happened. Prediction requires the fairly concrete specification of alternatives. This chapter thus also offers the policy analysts' answer to the question of OPTN applicability by sketching possible applications to medical records and evidence-based surgery. Whether any others choose to pursue them, I believe these applications convey the potential for greater use of private rulemaking in medical governance.

References

Aaron, Henry J., William B. Schwartz, and Melissa Cox. 2005. *Can we say no? The challenge of rationing health care.* Washington, DC: Brookings Institution Press.

Abecassis, M. M. 2006. Financial outcomes in transplantation: A provider's perspective. *American Journal of Transplantation* 6 (6): 1257–63.

Abt Associates, Inc. 1990. *Evaluation of the organ procurement and transplantation network: Final report.* Cambridge, MA: ABT Associates, Inc.

Ahearne, John, and Peter Blair. 2003. Expanding the use of the National Academies. In *Science and Technology Advice for Congress,* ed. M. Granger Morgan and Jon M. Peha, 118–33. Washington, DC: Resources for the Future.

Aldrich, John. 1995. *Why parties?The origin and transformation of party politics in America.* Chicago: University of Chicago Press.

Allen, Douglas W. 1991. What are transaction costs? *Research in Law and Economics* 14:1–18.

Allison, Graham T. 1971. *Essence of decision: Explaining the Cuban missile crisis.* Boston, MA: Little, Brown.

Ansell, Chris, and Alison Gash. 2008. Collaborative governance in theory and practice. *Journal of Public Administration Research and Theory* 18 (4): 543–71.

Arrow, Kenneth J. 1951. *Social choice and individual values.* New York: John Wiley & Sons.

———. 1963. Uncertainty and the welfare economics of medical care. *American Economic Review* 53 (5): 941–73.

———. 1972. Gifts and exchanges. *Philosophy and Public Affairs* 1 (4): 343–62.

Arthur, Brian. 1994. *Increasing returns and path dependence in the economy.* Ann Arbor: University of Michigan Press.

Ash, Joan S., Paul N. Gorman, Veena Seshadri, and William R. Hersh. 2004. Computerized physician order entry in U.S. hospitals: Results of a 2002 survey. *Journal of the American Medical Informatics Association* 11 (2): 95–99.

Aspden, Philip, Julie Wolcott, J. Lyle Bootman, and Linda R. Cronenwett. 2007. *Preventing medical errors.* Washington, DC: Institute of Medicine.

Axelrod, Robert. 1982. *The evolution of cooperation.* New York: Basic Books.

Ayanian, John Z., Paul D. Cleary, Joel S. Weissman, and Arnold M. Epstein. 1999. The effects of patients' preferences on racial differences in access to renal transplantation. *New England Journal of Medicine* 341 (22): 1661–69.

Ayres, Ian, Laura G. Dooley, and Robert S. Gaston. 1993. Unequal racial access to kidney transplantation. *Vanderbilt Law Review* 46 (4): 805–63.

Baciu, Alina, Kathleen Stratton, and Sheila P. Burke, eds. 2007. *The future of drug safety: Protecting the health of the public.* Washington, DC: National Academy Press.

Balla, Steven J., and Benjamin M. Daniels. 2007. Information technology and public commenting on agency regulations. *Regulation & Governance* 1 (1): 46–67.

Balla, Steven J., and John R. Wright. 2001. Interest groups, advisory committees, and congressional control of the bureaucracy. *American Journal of Political Science* 45 (4): 799–812.

———. 2003. Consensual rule making and the time it takes to develop rules. In *Politics, policy, and organizations: Frontiers in the scientific study of bureaucracy,* ed. George A. Krause and Kenneth J. Meier, 187–206. Ann Arbor: University of Michigan Press.

Banks, Jeffrey S. 1995. The design of institutions: An agency theory perspective. In *Institutional design,* ed. David L. Weimer, 17–36. Boston, MA: Kluwer Academic.

Bardach, Eugene, and Robert Kagan. 1982. *Going by the book: The problem of regulatory unreasonableness.* Philadelphia: Temple University Press.

Barke, Richard. 1986. *Science, technology and public policy.* Washington, DC: CQ Press.

Beito, David T. 2000. *From mutual aid to the welfare state: Fraternal societies and social services, 1890–1967.* Chapel Hill: University of North Carolina Press.

Bendor, Jonathan, and Adam Meirowitz. 2004. Spatial models of delegation. *American Political Science Review* 98 (2): 293–310.

Benjamin, Martin, Carl Cohen, and Eugene Grochowski. 1994. What transplantation can teach us about health care reform. *New England Journal of Medicine* 330 (12): 858–60.

Bernat, J. L., A. M. D'Alessandro, F. K. Port, T. P. Bleck, S. O. Head, J. Medina, S. H. Rosenbaum, et al. 2006. Report of a national conference on donation after cardiac death. *American Journal of Transplantation* 6 (2): 281–91.

Bernstein, Marver H. 1955. *Regulating business by independent commission.* Princeton, NJ: Princeton University Press.

Bertelli, Anthony M., and Laurence E. Lynn Jr. 2006. *Madison's managers: Public administration and the Constitution.* Baltimore: Johns Hopkins University Press.

Bleiklie, Ivar, Malcolm L. Goggin, and Christine Rothmayr. 2004. *Comparative biomedical policy: Governing assisted reproductive technologies.* New York: Routledge.

Blumstein, James F. 1989. Government's role in organ transplantation policy. In *Organ transplantation policy: Issues and prospects,* ed. James F. Blumstein and Frank A. Sloan, 5–39. Durham, NC: Duke University Press.

Bodenheimer, Thomas. 1997. The Oregon health plan: Lessons for the nation, first of two parts. *New England Journal of Medicine* 337 (9): 651–55.

Brown, Trevor L., and Matthew Potoski. 2003. Managing contract performance: A transaction cost approach. *Journal of Policy Analysis and Management* 22 (2): 275–97.

Burdick, James F. 1996. Testimony. U.S. Department of Health and Human Services public hearing on liver allocation and organ donation. Bethesda, MD. December 10, 1996.

———. 2004. Letter to Walter Graham, executive director of the United Network for Organ Sharing, as director, Office of Transplantation. October 29, 2004.

Calabresi, Guido, and Philip Bobbitt. 1978. *Tragic choices.* New York: W. W. Norton.

Callender, C. O., P. V. Miles, and M. B. Hall. 2003. Experience with national minority organ tissue transplant education program in the United States. *Transplantation Proceedings* 35 (3): 1151–52.

Carey, Mary Agnes. 2000. Congress tries two paths to bypass administration's new organ allocation rules. *CQ Weekly* (April 8): 838.

Cave, Jonathan, and Stephen W. Salant. 1995. Cartel quotas under majority rule. *American Economic Review* 85 (1): 82–102.

Cheibub, Jose Antonio, and Fernando Limongi. 2002. Democratic institutions and regime survival: Parliamentary and presidential democracies reconsidered. *Annual Review of Political Science* 5:151–79.

Cheit, Ross E. 1990. *Setting safety standards: Regulation in the public and private sectors.* Berkeley: University of California Press.

Cherikh, Wida, and Yulin Cheng. 2007. Updated report on the national voluntary variance to allocate A_2/A_2B deceased donor kidneys to B candidates. Prepared for Minority Affairs Committee by the Research Department, February 23. Richmond, VA: United Network for Organ Sharing.

Cherry, Mark J. 2005. *Kidney for sale by owner: Human organs, transplantation, and the market.* Washington, DC: Georgetown University Press.

Childress, James F. 1989. Ethical criteria for procuring and distributing organs for transplantation. In *Organ transplantation policy: Issues and prospects,* ed. James F. Blumstein and Frank A. Sloan, 87–113. Durham, NC: Duke University Press.

Childress, James F., and Catharyn T. Livermore, eds. 2006. *Organ donation: Opportunities for action.* Washington, DC: National Academy Press.

Coase, Ronald. 1937. The nature of the firm. *Economica* 4 (16): 386–405.

———. 1960. The problem of social cost. *Journal of Law and Economics* 3 (1): 1–44.

Coglianese, Cary. 1997. Assessing consensus: The promise and performance of negotiated rulemaking. *Duke Law Review* 46 (6): 1255–1349.

Coglianese, Cary, and David Lazer. 2003. Management-based regulation: Prescribing private management to achieve public goals. *Law and Society Review* 37 (4): 691–730.

Collins, Harry, and Robert Evans. 2007. *Rethinking expertise.* Chicago: University of Chicago Press.

Constas, Helen. 1958. Max Weber's two conceptions of bureaucracy. *American Journal of Sociology* 63 (4): 400–9.

Cooper, Jeffrey T., L. Thomas Chin, Nancy R. Krieger, Luis A Fernandez, David P. Foley, Yolanda T. Becker, Jon S. Odorico, et al. 2004. Donation after cardiac death: The University of Wisconsin experience with renal transplantation. *American Journal of Transplantation* 4 (9): 1490–94.

Croley, Steven, and William Funk. 1997. The Federal Advisory Committee Act and good government. *Yale Journal on Regulation* 14 (2): 452–557.

Culyer, Anthony, Christopher McCabe, Andrew Briggs, Karl Claxton, Martin Buxton, Ron Akehurst, Mark Sculpher, and John Brazier. 2007. Searching for a threshold, not setting one: The role of the National Institute for Health and Clinical Excellence. *Journal of Health Services Research and Policy* 12 (1): 56–58.

Cutler, David M. 2004. *Your money or your life: Strong medicine for America's healthcare system.* New York: Oxford University Press.

Danovitch, Gabriel M., Bernard Cohen, and Jacqueline M. A. Smits. 2002. Waiting time or wasted time? The case for using time on dialysis to determine waiting time in the allocation of cadaveric kidneys. *American Journal of Transplantation* 9 (11): 891–93.

Daubert, Gail L. 1998. Politics, policies, and problems with organ transplantation: Government regulation needed to ration organs equitably. *Administrative Law Review* 50 (2): 459–89.

Davidoff, Frank. 2006. Sex, politics, and morality at the FDA: Reflections on the plan B decision. *The Hastings Center Report* 36 (2): 20–48.

DeFrances, Carol J., Christine A. Lucus, Verita C. Buie, and Aleksandr Golosinskiy. 2007. 2006 National Hospital discharge survey. *National Health Statistics*, no. 5. Hyattsville, MD: National Center for Health Statistics.

Delmonico, Francis L., and Walter K. Graham. 2006. Direction of the Organ Procurement and Transplantation Network and United Network for Organ Sharing regarding the oversight of live donor transplantation and solicitation of organs. *American Journal of Transplantation* 6 (1): 37–40.

Delmonico, Francis L., Paul E. Morrissey, George S. Lipkowitz, Jeffrey S. Stoff, Jonathan Himmelfarb, William Harmon, Martha Pavlkis, et al. 2004. Donor kidney exchanges. *American Journal of Transplantation* 4 (10): 1628–34.

Dennis, J. Michael. 1992. A review of centralized rule-making in American transplantation. *Transplantation Reviews* 6 (2): 130–37.

———. 1995. Scarce medical resources: Hemodialysis and kidney transplantation. In *Local Justice in America*, ed. Jon Elster, 81–151. New York: Russell Sage Founation.

Denny, Donald. 1983. How organs are distributed. *Hastings Center Report* 6 (1): 26–27.

Denton, Timothy A., and George A. Diamond. 1995. For goodness' sake: Expected therapeutic benefit as a basis for healthcare delivery. *Clinical Chemistry* 41 (5): 799–809.

Deyo, Richard A., Bruce M. Psaty, George Simon, Edward H. Wagner, and Gilbert S. Omenn. 1997. The messenger under attack: Intimidation of researchers by special-interest groups. *New England Journal of Medicine* 336 (16): 1176–80.

Diamond, George A., and Sanjay Kaul. 2008. The disconnect between practice guidelines and clinical practice: Stressed out. *Journal of the American Medical Association* 300 (15): 1817–19.

Dilger, Robert J., Randolph R. Moffitt, and Linda Struyk. 1997. Privatization of municipal services in America's largest cities. *Public Administration Review* 57 (1) 21–26.

Dominguez, Alex. 2008. Six receive kidneys in multiple transplant. *Associated Press*, April 8.

Dranove, David. 2003. *What's your life worth? Health care rationing.* Upper Saddle River, NJ: Prentice Hall.

Dunlop, John. 1976. The limits of legal compulsion. *Labor Law Journal* 27 (2): 67–74.

Dworkin, Gerald. 1994. Markets and morals: The case for organ sales. In *Morality, harm, and the law*, ed. Gerald Dworkin, 155–61. Boulder, CO: Westview Press.

Edwards, Erick B., and Ann Harper. 1996. Liver allocation policy in the United States: 1987–1996. Public Access File, Log No. 51. Committee on Organ Procurement and Transplantation Policy. Washington, DC: National Research Council.

Edwards, Erick B., John P. Roberts, Maureen A. McBride, James A. Schulak, and Lawrence G. Hunsicker. 1999. The effect of the volume of procedures at transplantation centers on mortality after liver transplantation. *New England Journal of Medicine* 341 (27): 2049–53.

Egan, Thomas M., and Robert M. Kotloff. 2005. Pro/con debate: Lung allocation should be based on medical urgency and transplant survival and not on waiting time. *Chest* 128 (1): 407–15.

Egan, Thomas M., S. Murray, R. T. Bustami, T. H. Shearon, K. P. McCullough, L. B. Edwards, M. A. Coke, et al. 2006. Development of a new lung allocation system in the United States. *American Journal of Transplantation* 6 (5 part 2): 1212–27.

Englesbe, Michael J., Yasser Ads, Joshua A. Cohn, Christopher J. Sonnenday, R. Lynch, Randall S. Sung, Shawn J. Pelletier, John D. Birkmeyer, and Jeffrey D. Punch. 2008. The effects of donor and recipient practices on transplant center finances. *American Journal of Transplantation* 8 (3): 586–92.

Epstein, Arnold M., John Z. Ayanian, Joseph H. Keogh, Susan J. Noonan, Nancy Armistead, Paul D. Cleary, Joel S. Weissman, et al. 2003. Racial disparities in access to renal transplantation. *New England Journal of Medicine* 343 (21): 1537–45.

Epstein, David, and Sharyn O'Halloran. 1999. *Delegating powers: A transaction cost politics approach to policy making under separation of powers.* New York: Cambridge University Press.

Etheredge, Lynn M. 2007. A rapid-learning health system: What would a rapid-learning health system look like, and how might we get there? *Heath Affairs* 26 (2): w107–18.

Ferguson, John H., and Charles R. Sherman. 2001. Panelists' views of 68 NIH Consensus Conferences. *International Journal of Technology Assessment in Health Care* 17 (94): 541–58.

Fiorina, Morris. 1982. Legislative choice of regulatory forms: Legal process or administrative process. *Public Choice* 39 (1): 33–66.

Forbes, Melissa, Carolyn J. Hill, and Laurence E. Lynn Jr. 2006. The logic of governance in health care delivery: An analysis of the empirical literature. In *Public services performance: Perspectives on measurement and management,* ed. George Boyne, Kenneth Meier, Laurence O'Toole Jr., and Richard Walker, 254–74. Cambridge: Cambridge University Press.

Forman, Lisa M., and Michael R. Lucy. 2001. Predicting the prognosis of chronic liver disease: An evolution from child to MELD. *Hepatology* 33 (2): 473–75.

Fox, Renee C., and Judith P. Swazey. 1974. *The courage to fail: A social view of organ transplantation and dialysis.* Chicago: University of Chicago Press.

Frankel, Martin J. 1997. Analysis of testimony and written comments: Federal Register notice, November 13, 1996 and Public Hearings, December 10–12, 1996, on organ allocation policies. Washington, DC: U.S. Department of Health and Human Services, Public Health Service, Division of Transplantation.

Freeman, Jody. 2000. The private role in public governance. *New York University Law Review* 75 (3): 543–675.

Freeman, Jody, and Laura Langbein. 2000. Regulatory negotiation and the legitimacy benefit. *NYU Environmental Law Journal* 9 (1): 60–151.

Freeman, Richard B., Ann M. Harper, and Erick B. Edwards. 2002. Redrawing organ distribution boundaries: Results of a computer-simulated analysis for liver transplantation. *Liver Transplantation* 8 (8): 559–666.

Freeman, Richard B., and Goran B. Klintmalm. 2006. It is time to re-think 'extended criteria.' *American Journal of Transplantation* 6 (10): 2225–27.

Freeman, Richard B., Richard J. Rohrer, Eliezer Katz, W. David Lewis, Roger Jenkins, A. Benedict Cosimi, Francis Delmonico, et al. 2001. Preliminary results of a liver allocation plan using a continuous medical severity score that de-emphasizes waiting time. *Liver Transplantation* 7 (3): 173–78.

Freidson, Eliot. 1970. *Profession of medicine: A study of the sociology of applied knowledge.* New York: Dodd, Mead.

Friedman, Robert. 1978. Representation in regulatory decision making: Scientific, industrial, and consumer inputs to the F.D.A. *Public Administration Review* 38 (3): 205–14.

Froomkin, A. Michael. 2000. Wrong turn in cyberspace: Using ICANN to route around the APA and the Constitution. *Duke Law Review* 50 (1): 17–186.

Furth, Susan L., Pushkal P. Garg, Alicia M. Neu, Wenke Hwang, Barbara A. Fivush, and Neil R. Powe. 2000. Racial differences in access to the kidney transplant waiting list for children and adolescents with end-stage renal disease. *Pediatrics* 106 (4): pt. 1, 756–61.

Gabel, Matthew J., and Charles R. Shipan. 2004. A social choice approach to expert consensus panels. *Journal of Health Economics* 23 (3): 543–64.

Gais, Thomas L., Mark A. Peterson, and Jack L. Walker. 1984. Interest groups, iron triangles and representative institutions in American national government. *British Journal of Political Science* 14 (2): 161–85.

Garland, Michael J. 1992. Rationing in public: Oregon's priority-setting methodology. In *Rationing America's medical care: The Oregon plan and beyond*, ed. Martin A. Strosberg, Joshua M. Wiener, Robert Baker, and I. Ann Fein, 37–59. Washington, DC: Brookings Institution Press.

Gaston, Robert S., Ian Ayres, Laura G. Dooley, and Arnold G. Diethelm. 1993. Racial equity in renal transplantation: The disparate impact of HLA-based allocation. *Journal of the American Medical Association* 270 (11): 1352–56.

Gaston, Robert S., Gabriel M. Danovitch, Patricia L. Adams, James J. Wynn, Robert M. Merion, Mark H. Deierhoi, Robert A. Metzger, et al. 2003. The report of a national conference on the wait list for kidney transplantation. *American Journal of Transplantation* 3 (7): 775–85.

Geier, Steven S. 2008. UNOS Histo Committee Issues. PowerPoint presentation provided by Geier to the author. March 18, 2008.

George, Alexander L., and Andrew Bennett. 2005. *Case studies and theory development in the social sciences*. Cambridge, MA: The MIT Press.

Gerber, Alan S., and Eric C. Patashnik. 2006. Sham surgery: The problem of inadequate medical evidence. In *Promoting the general welfare: American democracy and the political economy of government performance*, ed. Alan S. Gerber and Eric C. Patashnik, 43–73. Washington, DC: Brookings Institution Press.

Gerling, Kerstin, Hans Peter Grüner, Alexandra Kiel, and Elisabeth Schulte. 2005. Information acquisition and decision making in committees: A survey. *European Journal of Political Economy* 21 (3): 563–97.

Gerring, John. 2004. What is a case study and what is it good for? *American Political Science Review* 98 (2): 341–54.

———. 2008. The mechanistic worldview: Thinking inside the box. *British Journal of Political Science* 38 (1): 161–79.

Gilbert, James C., Lori Brigham, D. Scott Batty, Jr., and Robert M. Veatch. 2005. The nondirected living donor program: A model for cooperative donation, recovery and allocation of living donor kidneys. *American Journal of Transplantation* 5 (1): 167–74.

Gilmour, John B., and David E. Lewis. 2006. Does performance budgeting work? An examination of the Office of Management and Budget's PART scores. *Public Administration Review* 66 (5): 742–52.

Globerman, Steven, and Aidan R. Vining. 1996. A framework for evaluating the government contracting-out decision with an application to information technology. *Public Administration Review* 56 (6): 577–86.

Goodin, Robert E., and John S. Dryzek. 2006. Deliberative impacts: The macro-political uptake of mini-publics. *Politics and Society* 34 (2): 219–44.

Gormley, William T., Jr. 1983. Policy, politics, and public utility regulation. *American Journal of Political Science* 27 (1): 86–105.

Gormley, William T., Jr., and David L. Weimer. 1999. *Organizational report cards.* Cambridge, MA: Harvard University Press.

Grantham, Dulcinia A. 2001. Transforming transplantation: The effect of the Health and Human Services Final Rule on the organ allocation system. *University of San Francisco Law Review* 35 (4): 751–82.

Gray, Bradford H., Michael K. Gusmano, and Sara R. Collins. 2003. AHCPR and the changing politics of health services research. *Health Affairs* Web exclusive (W3): 283–307.

Greenstein, S. M., R. Schechner, D. Senitzer, P. Louis, F. J. Veith, and V. A. Tellis. 1989. Does kidney distribution based upon HLA matching discriminate against blacks? *Transplantation Proceedings* 21 (6): 3874–75.

Grogan, Collen M., and Michael K. Gusmano. 2005. Deliberative democracy in theory and practice: Connecticut's Medicaid managed care council. *State Politics and Policy Quarterly* 5 (2): 126–46.

Gunningham, Neil, and Joseph Rees. 1997. Industry self-regulation: An institutional perspective. *Law and Policy* 19 (4): 363–414.

Guston, David. 2000. *Between politics and science: Assuring the integrity and productivity of research.* New York: Cambridge University Press.

Hacker, Jacob S. 1997. *The road to nowhere: The genesis of President Clinton's plan for health security.* Princeton, NJ: Princeton University Press.

Hardin, Russell. 1982. *Collective action.* Baltimore: Johns Hopkins University Press.

Harper, Ann M., Sarah E. Taranto, Erick B. Edwards, and O. Patrick Daily. 2000. An update on a successful simulation project: The UNOS liver allocation model. In *Proceedings of the 2000 Winter Simulation Conference*, ed. J. A. Jones, R. R. Barton, K. Kang, and P. A. Fishwick, 1955–62. Piscataway, NJ: Institute of Electrical and Electronics Engineers.

Harter, Philip. 1982. Negotiating regulations: A cure for malaise. *Georgetown Law Journal* 71 (1): 1–118.

Harvard Medical School. 1968. A definition of irreversible coma: Report of the ad hoc committee of the Harvard Medical School to examine the definition of brain death. *Journal of the American Medical Association* 205 (6): 85–88.

Hata, Yoshinobu, J. Michael Cecka, Steven Takemoto, Miyuki Ozawa, Yong W. Cho, and Paul I. Terasaki. 1998. Effects of changes in the criteria for nationally shared kidney transplants for HLA-matched patients. *Transplantation* 65 (2): 208–12.

Hauboldt, Richard H., and Seven G. Hanson. 2008. 2008 U.S. organ and tissue transplant cost estimates and discussion. Milliman Research Report. Brookfield, WI: Milliman.

Havighurst, Clark C. 1994. Forward: The place of private accrediting among the instruments of government. *Law and Contemporary Problems* 57 (4): 1–13.

Healy, Kieran. 2006. *Last best gifts: Altruism and the market for human blood and organs.* Chicago: University of Chicago Press.

Hodge, Graeme A. 2000. *Privatization: An international perspective.* Boulder, CO: Westview Press.

Hoffman, Sharona, and Andy Podgurski. 2008. Finding a cure: The case for regulation and oversight of electronic health record systems. *Harvard Journal of Law & Technology* 22 (1): 103–65.

Hollings, Robert, and Christal Pike-Nase. 1997. *Professional and occupational licensure in the United States.* Westport, CT: Greenwood Press.

Holmstrom, Bengt, and Jean Tirole. 1989. The theory of the firm. In *Handbook of Industrial Organization,* vol. 1, ed. Richard Schmalensee and Robert D. Willig, 61–133. New York: North-Holland.

Huber, John D., and Charles R. Shipan. 2002. *Deliberate discretion: The institutional foundations of bureaucratic autonomy.* New York: Cambridge University Press.

Huyse, Luc, and Stephen Parmentier. 1990. Decoding codes: The dialogue between consumers and suppliers through codes of conduct in the European community. *Journal of Consumer Policy* 13 (3): 253–72.

Institute of Medicine (IOM). 1999. *Organ procurement and transplantation: Assessing current policies and the potential impact of the DHHS Final Rule.* Washington, DC: National Academy Press.

———. 2001. *Crossing the quality chasm: A new health system for the 21st century.* Washington, DC: National Academy Press.

Islam, Roumeen. 2006. Does more transparency go along with better governance? *Economics and Politics* 18 (2): 121–67.

Jackman, Jennifer. 2002. Anatomy of a feminist victory: Winning the transfer of RU 486 patent rights to the United States, 1988–1994. *Women and Politics* 24 (3): 81–99.

Jacobs, Lawrence, Theodore Marmor, and Jonathan Oberlander. 1999. The Oregon health plan and the political paradox of rationing: What advocates and critics have claimed and what Oregon did. *Journal of Health Politics, Policy and Law* 24 (1): 161–80.

Jaffe, Louis. 1937. Law making by private groups. *Harvard Law Review* 51 (2): 201–53.

Jasanoff, Sheila. 1990. *The fifth branch: Science advisors as policymakers.* Cambridge, MA: Harvard University Press.

———. 1995. *Science at the bar: Law, science, and technology in America.* Cambridge, MA: Harvard University Press.

Jensen, Michael, C., and William H. Meckling. 1976. Theory of the firm: Managerial behavior, agency costs, and ownership structure. *Journal of Financial Economics* 3 (4): 305–60.

Johnson, Stephen M. 1998. The Internet changes everything: Revolutionizing public participation and access to government information through the Internet. *Administrative Law Review* 50 (2): 277–337.

Jones, Bryan D., and Frank R. Baumgartner. 2005. *The politics of attention: How government prioritizes problems.* Chicago: University of Chicago Press.

Jost, Timothy Stoltzfus. 1983. The Joint Commission on Accreditation of Hospitals: Private regulation of health care and the public interest. *Boston College Law Review* 24 (4): 835–923.

Kahneman, Daniel, and Amos Tversky. 1984. Choices, values and frames. *American Psychologist* 39 (4): 341–50.

Kamath, Patrick S., Russel H. Wiesner, Michael Malinchoc, Walter Kremers, Termmy M. Therneau, Catherine L. Kosberg, Gennardo D'Amico, E. Rolland Dickson, and W. Ray Kim. 2001. A model to predict survival in patients with end-stage liver disease. *Hepatology* 33 (2): 464–70.

Kaplan, Robert M. 1992. A quality-of-life approach to health resource allocation. In *Rationing America's medical care: The Oregon plan and beyond,* ed. Martin A. Strosberg, Martin A., Joshua M. Wiener, Robert Baker, and I. Ann Fein, 60–77. Washington, DC: Brookings Institution Press.

Karkkainen, Bradley C. 2006. Information enforcing environmental regulation. *Florida State Law Review* 33 (3): 861–62.

Kaserman, David L., and A. H. Barnett. 2002. *The U.S. organ procurement system: A prescription for reform.* Washington, DC: American Enterprise Institute for Public Policy Research.

Kaufman, Herbert. 1960. *The forest ranger: A study in administrative behavior.* Baltimore: Johns Hopkins University Press.

Keith, Douglas, Valerie B. Ashby, Friedrich K. Port, and Alan B. Leichtman. 2008. Insurance type and minority status associated with large disparities in prelisting dialysis among candidates for kidney transplantation. *Clinical Journal of the American Society of Nephrology* 3 (2): 463–70.

Kilner, John F. 1990. *Who lives? Who dies? Ethical criteria in patient selection.* New Haven, CN: Yale University Press.

Kingdon, John W. 1984. *Agendas, alternatives, and public policies.* Boston, MA: Little Brown.

Klassen, Ann C., David K. Klassen, Ron Brokmeyer, Richard G. Frank, and Katherine Marconi. 1998. Factors influencing waiting time and successful receipt of cadaveric liver transplant in the United States, 1990 to 1992. *Medical Care* 36 (3): 281–94.

Knill, Christopher, and Dirk Lehmkuhl. 2002. Private actors and the state: Internationalization and changing patterns of governance. *Governance* 15 (1): 41–63.

Kohn, Linda T., Janet M. Corrigan, and Molla S. Donaldson. 2000. *To err is human: Building a safer health system.* Washington, DC: Institute of Medicine.

Kopans, Daniel B. 1999. The breast cancer screening controversy and the National Institutes of Health consensus development conference on breast cancer screening for women ages 40–49. *Radiology* 210 (11): 4–9.

Laffell, Mary S., and Andrea A. Zachary. 1999. The national impact of the 1995 changes to the UNOS renal allocation system. *Clinical Transplantation* 13 (4): 287–95.

Langbein, Laura I., and Cornelius M. Kerwin. 2000. Regulatory negotiation versus conventional rule making: Claims, counterclaims, and empirical evidence. *Journal of Public Administration Research and Theory* 10 (3): 599–632.

La Puma, John. 1992. Quality-adjusted life-years: Why physicians should reject Oregon's plan. In *Rationing America's medical care: The Oregon plan and beyond*, ed. Martin A. Strosberg, Joshua M. Wiener, Robert Baker, and I. Ann Fein, 125–31. Washington, DC: Brookings Institution Press.

Laugesen, Miriam J. 2009. Siren song: Physicians, Congress, and Medicare fees. *Journal of Health Politics, Policy and Law* 34 (2): 157–79.

Laurie, Peter, Cristina M. Almeida, Nicholas Stine, Alexander R. Stine, and Sindney M. Wolfe. 2006. Financial conflict of interest disclosure and voting patterns at Food and Drug Administration Drug Advisory Committee meetings. *Journal of the American Medical Association* 295 (16): 1921–28.

Lavertu, Stéphane, and David L. Weimer. 2008. Information costs, policy uncertainty, and political control: Federal advisory committees at the FDA. Mimeo.

Lazda, V. A. 1991. An evaluation of a local variance of the United Network for Organ Sharing (UNOS) point system on the distribution of cadaver kidneys to waiting minority recipients. *Transplantation Proceedings* 23 (1): 901–2.

Lazda, V. A., and M. E. Blaesing. 1989. Is allocation of kidneys on the basis of HLA match equitable in multiracial populations? *Transplantation Proceedings* 21 (1): 1415–16.

Leavitt, Michael. 2007. Statement. American Health Information Community Successor Public Information Meeting, Washington, DC.

Leichter, Howard M. 1999. Oregon's bold experiment: Whatever happened to rationing? *Journal of Health Politics, Policy and Law* 24 (1): 147–60.

———. 2004. Obstacles to dependent health care access in Oregon: Health insurance or health care? *Journal of Health Politics, Policy and Law* 29 (2): 237–68.

Lin, Grace A., R. Adam Dudley, F. L. Lucas, David J. Malenka, Eric Vittinghoff, and Rita F. Redberg. 2008. Frequency of stress testing to document ischemia prior to elective percutaneous coronary intervention. *Journal of the American Medical Association* 300 (15): 1765–73.

Lomas, Jonathan. 1991. Words without action? The production, dissemination, and impact of consensus recommendations. *Annual Review of Public Health* 12:41–64.

Lowi, Theodore J. 1969. *The end of liberalism.* New York: W. W. Norton.

Lynn, Laurence E. Jr., Carolyn J. Heinrich, and Carolyn J. Hill. 2000. Studying governance and public management: Why? How? in *Governance and performance: New perspectives,* ed. Carolyn J. Heinrich and Laurence E. Lynn Jr., 1–33. Washington, DC: Georgetown University Press.

———. 2001. *Improving governance: A new logic for empirical research.* Washington, DC: Georgetown University Press.

Lyons, Bruce R. 1995. Specific investments, economies of scale, and the make-or-buy decision: A test of transaction cost theory. *Journal of Economic Behavior and Organization* 26 (3): 431–43.

Macher, Jeffrey T., and Barak D. Richman. 2008. Transaction cost economics: An assessment of the empirical research in the social sciences. *Business and Politics* 10 (1): 1.

Majone, Giandomenico. 1996. *Regulating Europe.* London: Routledge.

Marchione, Marilynn. 1999. Compromise reached in organ-sharing feud: Illinois agrees to 'paybacks' to limit exports from Wisconsin. *Milwaukee Journal Sentinel* July 30, 1.

Markle, Gerald E., and Daryl E. Chubin. 1987. Consensus development in biomedicine: The liver transplant controversy. *Milbank Quarterly* 65 (1): 1–24.

Marmor, Ted, Richard Freeman, and Kieke Okma. 2005. Comparative perspectives and policy learning in the world of health care. *Journal of Comparative Policy Analysis* 7 (4): 331–48.

Marshall, C. Kevin. 2007. Memorandum for Daniel Meron, general counsel, U.S. Department of Health and Human Services. Re.: Legality of alternative organ donation practices under 42 U.S.C. Section 274e. March 28. Washington, DC: U.S. Department of Justice, Office of the Deputy Assistant Attorney General.

Matsuoka, L., T. Shah, S. Aswad, S. Bunnapradist, Y. Cho, R. G. Mendez, R. Medez, and R. Selby. 2006. Pulsatile perfusion reduces the incidence of delayed graft function in expanded criteria donor kidney transplantation. *American Journal of Transplantation* 6 (6): 1473–78.

Mayes, Rick, and Robert A. Berenson. 2006. *Medicare prospective payment and the shaping of U.S. health care.* Baltimore: Johns Hopkins University Press.

McAfee, R. Preston, and John McMillian. 1996. Analyzing the airwaves auction. *Journal of Economic Perspectives* 10 (1): 159–75.

McCubbins, Mathew D., Roger G. Noll, and Barry R. Weingast. 1987. Administrative procedures as instruments of political control. *Journal of Law, Economics, and Organization* 3 (2): 243–77.

————. 1989. Structure and process, politics and policy: Administrative arrangements and the political control of agencies. *Virginia Law Review* 75 (2): 431–82.

McCubbins, Mathew D., and Thomas Schwartz. 1984. Congressional oversight overlooked: Police patrols versus fire alarms. *American Journal of Political Science* 28 (1): 165–79.

McKenna, Rachel M., and Steven K. Takemoto. 2000. Improving HLA matching for kidney transplantation by use of CREGs. *The Lancet* 355 (9218): 1842–43.

McMullen, Laura E. 1999. Equitable allocation of human organs: An examination of the new federal regulation. *Journal of Legal Medicine* 20 (3): 405–24.

Mechanic, David. 1998. The functions and limitations of trust in the provision of medical care. *Journal of Health Politics, Policy and Law* 23 (4): 661–86.

Medicare Payment Advisory Commission. 2008. *Report to the Congress: Medicare payment policy.* March. Washington, DC: MedPAC.

Meier, Kenneth J., and Laurence J. O'Toole. 2006. *Bureaucracy in a democratic state: A governance perspective.* Baltimore: Johns Hopkins University Press.

Mendeloff, John. 1979. *Regulating safety: An economic and political analysis of occupational safety and health policy.* Cambridge, MA: MIT Press.

Mendeloff, John, Kilkon Ko, Mark S. Roberts, Margaret Byrne, and Mary Amanda Dew. 2004. Procuring organ donors as a health investment: How much should we be willing to spend? *Transplantation* 78 (12): 1704–710.

Mesich-Brant, Jennifer L., and Lawrence J. Grossback. 2005. Assisting altruism: Evaluating legally binding consent in organ donation policy. *Journal of Health Politics, Policy and Law* 30 (4): 687–717.

Metzger, Robert A., Francis L. Delmonico, Sandy Feng, Friedrich K. Port, James J. Wynn, and Robert M. Merion. 2003. Expanded criteria donors for kidney transplantation. *American Journal of Transplantation* 3 (Supplement 4): 114–25.

Miller, Gary J., and Andrew B. Whitford. 2006. The principal's moral hazard: Constraints on the use of incentives within hierarchy. *Journal of Public Administration Research and Theory* 17 (2): 213–33.

Miller, Mark E. 2007. Producing comparative-effectiveness information. Statement before the Subcommittee on Health, Committee on Ways and Means, U.S. House of Representatives, June 12. Washington, DC: Medicare Payment Advisory Commission. www.medpac.gov/documents/061207_WandM_Testimony _MedPAC_CE.pdf.

Miller, Nancy A, Sarah Ramsland, and Charlene Harrington. 1999. Trends and issues in the Medicaid 1915(c) Waiver Program. *Health Care Financing Review* 20 (4): 139–60.

Mone, Thomas D. 2002. The business of organ procurement. *Current Opinions in Organ Transplantation* 7 (1): 60–64.

Moore, W. John. 1998. Life-and-death lobbying. *National Journal* 30 (28): 631.

Morgan, M. Granger, and Jon M. Peha. 2003. *Science and technology advice for Congress.* Washington, DC: Resources for the Future.

Morrissey, Joseph P., Mark Tausig, and Michael Lindsey. 1985. Community mental health delivery systems: A network perspective. *American Behavioral Scientist* 28 (5): 704–20.

Moseley, J. Bruce, Kimberly O'Malley, Nancy J. Peterson, Terri J. Menke, Baruch A. Brody, David H. Kuykendall, John C. Hollingsworth, Carol M. Ashton, and Nelda P. Wray. 2002. A controlled trial of arthroscopic surgery for osteoarthritis of the knee. *New England Journal of Medicine* 347 (2): 81–88.

Murphy, Timothy F. 2004. Gaming the transplant system. *American Journal of Bioethics* 4 (1): W28.

Mykhalovskiy, Eric, and Lorna Weir. 2004. The problem of evidence-based medicine: Directions for social science. *Social Science & Medicine* 59 (5): 1059–69.

National Center for Health Statistics. 2007. *Health, United States, 2007 with chartbook on trends in the health of Americans.* Washington, DC: U.S. Government Printing Office.

National Conference of Commissioners on Uniform State Laws. 1980. Uniform Determination of Death Act. Philadelphia: NCCUSL Archives, University of Pennsylvania Law School. http://www.law.upenn.edu/bll/archives/ulc/fnact99/1980s/udda80.pdf.

———. 2008. Uniform Anatomical Gift Act. http://www.anatomicalgiftact.org.

National Institute for Health and Clinical Excellence (NICE). 2005. *A guide to NICE.* London. April. http://www.nice.org.uk.

National Institute of Medicine. 1997. Breast cancer screening for women ages 40–49. *NIH Consensus Statement Online* 15 (1): 1–35.

Nelson, Paul W., Michael D. Landreneau, Alan M. Luger, George E. Pierce, Gilbert Ross, Charles F. Shield, Bradley A. Warady, et al. 1998. Ten-year experience in transplantation of A_2 kidneys into B and O recipients. *Transplantation* 65 (2): 256–60.

Neumann, Peter J. 2005. *Using cost-effectiveness analysis to improve health care: Opportunities and barriers.* New York: Oxford University Press.

Nonet, Phillippe, and Philip Selznick. 1978. *Law and society in transition: Toward responsive law.* New York: Harper and Row.

Nord, Erik. 1993. Unjustified use of the quality of well-being scale in priority setting in Oregon. *Health Policy* 24 (1): 45–53.

Oberlander, Jonathan, Theodore Marmor, and Lawrence Jacobs. 2001. Rationing medical care: Rhetoric and reality in the Oregon health plan. *Canadian Medical Association Journal* 164 (11): 1583–87.

Office of Inspector General. 1991. *The distribution of organs for transplantation: Expectations and practices.* Washington, DC: U.S. Department of Health and Human Services.

Oliver, Thomas R. 1993. Analysts, advice, and congressional leadership: The Physician Payment Review Commission and the politics of medicare. *Journal of Health Politics, Policy and Law* 18 (1): 113–74.

Oliver, Thomas R., and Rachel Friedman Singer. 2006. Health services research as a source of legislative analysis and input: The role of the California Health Benefits Review Program. *Health Services Research* 41 (3 pt 2): 1124–58.

Olsen, Leigh Anne, Dara Aisner, and J. Michael McGinnis, eds. 2007. *The learning healthcare system.* Washington, DC: National Academies Press.

Oregon Health Services Commission. 2005. *Prioritization of health services: A report to the governor and 73rd Oregon legislative assembly.* Salem, OR: Department of Administrative Services.

Organ Procurement and Transplantation Network (OPTN). 2005. Interim report: Policy Oversight Committee, December 14. Richmond, VA: United Network for Organ Sharing.

———. 2007. *Policies.* Washington, DC: U.S. Department of Health and Human Services. http://optn.transplant.hrsa.gov/policiesAndBylaws/policies.asp.

———. 2008a. *Kidney allocation concepts: Request for information.* Kidney Transplantation Committee, September 24. Richmond, VA: United Network for Organ Sharing.

———. 2008b. *Proposed national system for the allocation of deceased donor kidneys.* Kidney Transplantation Committee, March 1. Richmond, VA: United Network for Organ Sharing.

———. 2009. Data reports: National data. Washington, DC: U.S. Department of Health and Human Services. http://optn.transplant.hrsa.gov/data/.

Organ Procurement and Transplantation Network/Scientific Registry of Transplant Recipients (OPTN/SRTR). 2005. *Annual report.* Washington, DC: U.S. Department of Health and Human Services.

Ostrom, Elinor. 1990. *Governing the commons: The evolution of institutions for collective action.* New York: Cambridge University Press.

Page, Scott E. 2006. Path dependence. *Quarterly Journal of Political Science* 1 (1): 87–115.

Pearson, Steven D., and Michael D. Rawlins. 2005. Quality, innovation, and value for money: NICE and the British National Health Service. *Journal of the American Medical Association* 294 (20): 2618–22.

Petracca, Mark. 1986. Federal advisory committees, interest groups, and the administrative state. *Congress & The Presidency* 13 (1): 83–114.

Physician Payment Review Commission. 1997. *Annual report to Congress.* Washington, DC: Physician Payment Review Commission.

Pickering, Larry K. 2002. Development of pediatric vaccine recommendations and policies. *Seminars in Pediatric Infectious Diseases* 13 (3): 148–54.

Pierce, Gene A., and John C. McDonald. 1996. UNOS history. In *UNOS organ procurement, preservation, and distribution in transplantation*, ed. Michael C. Phillips, 1–5. Richmond, VA: United Network for Organ Sharing.

Pierson, Paul. 2000. Path dependence, increasing returns, and the study of politics. *American Political Science Review* 94 (2): 251–67.

Plante, Charles L. 2000. 1971 Medicare amendment: Reflection on the passage of the end-stage renal disease medicare program. *American Journal of Kidney Diseases* 35 (4): S45-48.

Porter, Michael E., and Elizabeth Olmsted Teisberg. 2006. *Redefining health care: Creating value-based competition on results.* Boston, MA: Harvard Business School Press.

Portnoy, Barry, Jennifer Miller, Kathryn Brown-Huamani, and Emily DeVoto. 2007. Impact of the National Institutes of Health Consensus Development Program on stimulating National Institutes of health-funded research, 1998 to 2001. *International Journal of Technology Assessment in Health Care* 23 (3): 343–48.

Powell, G. Bingham. 2000. *Elections as instruments of democracy: Majoritarian and proportional visions.* New Haven, CT: Yale University Press.

Prendergast, Canice. 1999. The provision of incentives in firms. *Journal of Economic Literature* 37 (1): 7–63.

President. 2004. Executive Order 13335—Incentives for the use of health information technology and establishing the position of the national health information technology coordinator. *Federal Register* 69, no. 84 (2004): 24059–61.

President's Commission for the Study of Ethical Problems in Medicine and Biomedical and Behavioral Research. 1981. *Defining death: A report on the medical, legal and ethical issues in the determination of death.* Washington, DC: U.S. Government Printing Office.

Pressman, Jeffrey L., and Aaron Wildavsky. 1973. *Implementation.* Berkeley: University of California Press.

Prottas, Jeffrey. 1994. *The most useful gift: Altruism and the public policy of organ transplants.* San Francisco, CA: Jossey-Bass.

Provan, Keith G., Amy Fish, and Joerg Sydow. 2007. Interorganizational networks at the network level: A review of the empirical literature on whole networks. *Journal of Management* 33 (3): 479–516.

Provan, Keith G., and Patrick Kenis. 2008. Modes of network governance: Structure, management, and effectiveness. *Journal of Public Administration Research and Theory* 18 (2): 229–52.

Provan, Keith G., and H. Brinton Milward. 1995. A preliminary theory of interorganizational network effectiveness: A comparative study of four community health systems. *Administrative Science Quarterly* 40 (1): 1–33.

Rabkin, John M. 1999. Geographic favoritism in liver transplantation. *New England Journal of Medicine* 340 (12): 964.

Ransohoff, David F., and Russell P. Harris. 1997. Lessons form the mammography screening controversy: Can we improve the debate. *Annals of Internal Medicine* 127 (11): 1029–34.

Rapaport, Felix T. 1986. The case for a living emotionally related international kidney donor exchange registry. *Transplantation Proceedings* 18 (2): 5–9.

Rees, Joseph V. 2008. The orderly use of experience: Pragmatism and the development of hospital industry self-regulation. *Regulation & Governance* 2 (1): 9–29.

Resnick, Andrew S., Diane Corrigan, James L. Mullen, and Larry R. Kaiser. 2005. Surgeon contribution to hospital bottom line: Not all are created equal. *Annals of Surgery* 242 (4): 530–39.

Rettig, Richard A. 1982. The federal government and social planning for end-stage renal disease: Past, present, and future. *Seminars in Nephrology* 2 (2): 111–33.

———. 1989. The politics of organ transplantation: A parable of our time. *Journal of Health Politics, Policy and Law* 14 (1): 191–227.

———. 1991. Origins of the medicare kidney disease entitlement: The Social Security amendments of 1972. In *Biomedical politics*, ed. Kathi E. Hanna, 176–208. Washington, DC: National Academy Press.

Rettig, Richard, Laurence Early, and Richard Merrill, eds. 1992. *Food and Drug Advisory Committees.* Washington, DC: National Academy Press.

Riker, William H., and Itai Sened. 1991. A positive theory of the origin of property rights: Airport slots. *American Journal of Political Science* 35 (4): 951–69.

Riker, William H., and David L. Weimer. 1995. The political economy of transformation: Liberalization and property rights. In *Modern political economy: Old topics, new directions.*, ed. Jeffrey Banks and Eric Hanushek, 80–107. New York: Cambridge University Press.

Rivlin, Alice M. 1983. An intelligent politician's guide to dealing with experts. *Commencement Addresses, 1974–1995.* Santa Monica, CA: The RAND Graduate School.

Rivlin, Alice M., and Joseph R. Antos, eds. 2007. *Restoring fiscal sanity 2007: The health spending challenge.* Washington, DC: Brookings Institution Press.

Roberts, Alasdair. 2006. *Blacked out: Government secrecy in the information age.* New York: Cambridge University Press.

Roberts, James S., Jack G. Coate, and Robert R. Redman. 1987. A history of the joint commission on accreditation of hospitals. *Journal of the American Medical Association* 258 (7): 10–14.

Rohr, John A. 1980. Ethics for the senior executive service. *Administration and Society* 12 (2): 203–16.

Rohrer, Richard J. 1996. Prepared testimony, public hearings on liver allocation and organ donation. December 10–13, 1996. Bethesda, MD: U.S. Department of Health and Human Services.

Rosenbloom, David H. 2000. *Building a legislative-centered public administration: Congress and the administrative state, 1946–1999.* Tuscaloosa: University of Alabama Press.

Rosengard, Bruce R., Sandy Feng, Edward J. Alfrey, Jonathan G. Zaroff, Jean C. Edmond, Mitchell L. Henrey, Edward R. Garrity, et al. 2002. Report of the crystal city meeting to maximize the use of organs recovered from the cadaver donor. *American Journal of Transplantation* 2 (8): 701–11.

Ross, Laine Friedman, David T. Rubin, Mark Siegler, Michelle A. Josephson, J. Richard Thistlethwaite Jr., and E. Steve Woodle. 1997. Ethics of a paired-kidney-exchange program. *New England Journal of Medicine* 336 (24): 1752–55.

Ross, Lainie Friedman, and Stefanos Zenios. 2004. Practical and ethical challenges to paired exchange programs. *American Journal of Transplantation* 4 (10): 1553–54.

Ross, Stephen A. 1973. The economic theory of agency: The principal's problem. *American Economic Review* 63 (2): 134–39.

Russo, C. Allison, Pamela Owens, Claudia Steiner, and Justin Josephsen. 2007. *Ambulatory surgery in U.S. hospitals, 2003—HCUP fact book no. 9.* Rockville, MD: Agency for Healthcare Research and Quality. www.ahrq.gov/data/hcup/factbk9/.

Sackett, David L., William M. C. Rosenberg, J. A. Muir Gray, R. Brain Haynes, and W. Scott Richardson. 1996. Evidence-based medicine: What it is and what it isn't. *British Medical Journal* 312 (7023): 71–72.

Saidman, Susan L., Alvin E. Roth, Tayfun Sönmez, M. Utku Ünver, and Francis L. Delmonico. 2006. Increasing the opportunity of live kidney donation by matching for two- and three-way exchanges. *Transplantation* 81 (5): 773–82.

Sappington, David E. M. 1991. Incentives in principal-agent relationships. *Journal of Economic Perspectives* 5 (2): 45–66.

Schlander, Michael. 2007. *Health technology assessments by the National Institute for Health and Clinical Excellence.* New York: Springer.

Schlesinger, Mark. 2002. A loss of faith: The sources of reduced political legitimacy for the American medical profession. *Milbank Quarterly* 80 (2): 185–235.

Schneider, Saundra K. 1997. Medicaid section 1115 waivers: Shifting health care reform to the states. *Publius* 27 (2): 89–109.

Schold, J. D., R. J. Howard, M. J. Scicchitano, and H. U. Meier-Kriesche. 2006. The expanded criteria donor policy: An evaluation of program objectives and indirect ramifications. *American Journal of Transplantation* 6 (7): 1689–95.

Schotter, Andrew. 1981. *The economic theory of social institutions.* New York: Cambridge University Press.

Schreiner, George E. 2000. How end-stage renal disease (ESRD)–Medicare developed. *American Journal of Kidney Diseases* 35 (4): S37-44.

Schwindt, Richard, and Aidan R. Vining. 1986. Proposal for a future delivery market for transplant organs. *Journal of Health Politics, Policy and Law* 11 (3): 483–500.

Scientific Registry of Transplant Recipients (SRTR). 2008. Integrating a measure of life years from transplant (LYFT) into deceased donor kidney allocation. PowerPoint presentation to Minority Affairs Committee, February 1. Richmond, VA: United Network for Organ Sharing.

Segev, Dorry L., Sommer E. Gentry, Daniel S. Warren, Brigitte Reeb, and Robert A. Montgomery. 2005. Kidney paired donation and optimizing the use of live donor organs. *Journal of the American Medical Association* 293 (15): 1883–90.

Selznick, Philip. 1949. *TVA and grass roots.* Berkeley: University of California Press.

Shafer, Teresa J., Dennis Wagner, John Chessare, Francis A. Zampiello, Virginia McBride, and Jude Perdue. 2006. Organ donation breakthrough collaborative: Increasing organ donation through system redesign. *Critical Care Nurse* 26 (2): 33–48.

Sheehy, Ellen, Suzanne L. Conrad, Lori E. Brigham, Richard Luskin, Phyllis Weber, Mark Eakin, Lawrence Schkade, and Lawrence Hunsicket. 2003. Estimating the number of potential organ donors in the United States. *New England Journal of Medicine* 349 (7): 667–74.

Shelanski, Howard A., and Peter G. Klein. 1995. Empirical evidence in transaction cost economics: A review and assessment. *Journal of Law, Economics, and Organization* 11 (2): 335–61.

Sheldon, Trevor A., Nicky Cullum, Diane Dawson, Annette Lankshear, Karin Lowson, Ian Watt, Peter West, Dianne Wright, and John Wright. 2004. What's the evidence that NICE guidance has been implemented? Results from a national evaluation using time series analysis, audit of patients' notes, and interviews. *British Medical Journal* 329 (7473): 999–1006.

Shepard, Lawrence. 1986. Cartelization of the California-Arizona orange industry, 1934–1981. *Journal of Law and Economics* 29 (1): 83–123.

Shimazono, Yosuke. 2007. The state of international organ trade: A provisional picture based on integration of available information. *Bulletin of the World Health Organization* 85 (12): 955–61.

Shuck, Peter. 1979. Litigation, bargaining, and regulation. *Regulation* 3 (4): 26–34.

Slater, Gary, and David A. Spencer. 2000. The uncertain foundations of transaction costs economics. *Journal of Economic Issues* 34 (1): 61–87.

Smith, Bruce L. R. 1992. *The advisors: Scientists in the policy process.* Washington, DC: Brookings Institution Press.

Smith, David G. 1992. *Paying for Medicare: The politics of reform.* New York: Aldine.

Smith, Jean C. 2008. Assistant to the director for Immunization Policy, Centers for Disease Control and Prevention, e-mail communication with Stéphane Lavertu. July 24, 2008.

Smith, Jean C., Dixie E. Snider, and Larry K. Pickering. 2009. Immunization policy development in the United States: The role of the Advisory Committee on Immunization Practices. *Annals of Internal Medicine* 150 (1): 45–49.

Spence, A. Michael, and Richard Zeckhauser. 1971. Insurance, information, and individual action. *American Economic Review* 61 (2): 380–87.

Spielman, Bethany. 2003. Should consensus be the 'commission method' in the US? The perspective of the Federal Advisory Committee Act, regulations, and case law. *Bioethics* 17 (4): 341–56.

Starzl, T. E., T. R. Hakala, A. Tzakis, R. Gordon, A. Strieber, L. Makowka, J. Klimoski, and H. T. Bahnson. 1987. A multifactoral system for equitable selection of cadaver kidney recipients. *Journal of the American Medical Association* 257 (22): 3037–75.

Starzl, T. E., R. Shapiro, and L. Teperman. 1989. The point system for organ distribution. *Transplantation Proceedings* 21 (3): 3432–36.

Steinbrook, Robert. 2004. Science, politics, and federal advisory committees. *New England Journal of Medicine* 350 (14): 1454–60.

Stevens, Rosemary A. 2001. Public roles for the medical profession in the United States: Beyond theories of decline and fall. *Milbank Quarterly* 79 (3): 327–53.

Stewart, Richard. 1975. The reformation of American administrative law. *Harvard Law Review* 88 (8): 1669–1813.

Stone, Deborah A. 2002. *The policy paradox: The art of political decision making.* New York: Norton.

Su, Zuanming, Stefanos A. Zenios, Harini Chakkera, Edgar L. Milford, and Glenn M. Chertow. 2004. Diminishing significance of HLA matching in kidney transplantation. *American Journal of Transplantation* 4 (9): 1501–8.

Sung, Randall S., Mary K. Guidinger, Craig D. Lake, Maureen A. McBride, Stuart M. Greenstein, Francis L. Delmonico, Friedrich K. Port, Robert M. Merion, and Alan B. Leichtman. 2005. Impact of the expanded criteria donor allocation system on the use of expanded criteria donor kidneys. *Transplantation* 79 (9): 1257–61.

Taranto, Sarah E., Ann M. Harper, Erick B. Edwards, John D. Rosendale, Maureen A. McBride, O. Patrick Daily, Dan Murphy, Bill Poos, Janet Reust, and Bruce Schmeiser. 2000. Developing a national allocation model for cadaveric kidneys. In *Proceedings of the 2000 Winter Simulation Conference*, ed. J. A. Jones, R. R. Barton, K. Kang, and P. A. Fishwick, 1971–77. New York: Association for Computing Machinery.

Task Force on Organ Transplantation. 1986. *Organ transplantation: Issues and recommendations.* Washington, DC: U.S. Department of Health and Human Services.

Taylor, James Stacey. 2005. *Stakes and kidneys: Why markets in human body parts are morally imperative.* Burlington, VT: Ashgate Publishing.

Taylor, Michael. 1982. *Community, anarchy, and liberty.* New York: Cambridge University Press.

Tenbensel, Tim. 2002. Interpreting public input into priority-setting: The role of mediating institutions. *Health Policy* 62 (2): 173–94.

Thompson, David, Larry Waisanen, Robert Wolfe, Robert M. Merion, Keith McCullough, and Ann Rodgers. 2004. Simulating the allocation of organs for transplantation. *Health Care Management Science* 7 (4): 331–38.

Thompson, Frank J., and Courtney Burke. 2007. Executive federalism and Medicaid demonstration waivers: Implications for policy and democratic process. *Journal of Health Politics, Policy and Law* 32 (6): 971–1004.

Tilney, Nicholas L. 2003. *Transplant: From myth to reality.* New Haven, CT: Yale University Press.

Titmuss, Richard. 1971. *The gift relationship: From human blood to social policy.* New York: Vintage.

Trubek, Louise G., Joseph V. Rees, A. Bryce Hoflund, Marybeth Farquhar, and Carol A. Heimer. 2008. Health care and new governance: The quest for effective regulation. *Regulation & Governance* 2 (1): 1–8.

Tuohy, Carolyn Hughes. 1999. *Accidental logics: The dynamics of change in the health care arena in the United States, Britain, and Canada.* New York: Oxford University Press.

Turcotte, Jeremiah G. 1999. Geographic favoritism in liver transplantation. *New England Journal of Medicine* 340 (12): 963.

Ubel, Peter A., Cindy L. Bryce, Laura A. Siminoff, Arthur L. Caplan, and Robert M. Arnold. 2000. Pennsylvania's voluntary benefits program: Evaluating an innovative proposal for increasing organ donation. *Health Affairs* 19 (5): 206–11.

Ubel, Peter A., and Arthur L. Caplan. 1998. Geographic favoritism in liver transplantation: Unfortunate for unfair? *New England Journal of Medicine* 339 (18): 1322–25.

UK Transplant. 1999. *Donor organ sharing scheme: Operating principles for liver transplantation units in the UK and the Republic of Ireland.* London: National Health Service.

United Network for Organ Sharing (UNOS). 1994a. Point change results from UNOS Study. *UNOS Update* (December):18.

———. 1994b. UNOS statement of principles and objectives of equitable organ allocation. Adopted by UNOS Board of Directors, June 29, 1994.

———. 2000. *2000 Annual report of the U.S. Scientific Registry of Transplant Recipients and the Organ Procurement and Transplant Network: Transplant data, 1990–1999.* Rockville, MD: U.S. Department of Health and Human Services.

———. 2001. Proposals for public comment, August 17, 2001. Richmond, VA: United Network for Organ Sharing.

———. 2002a. Allocation of livers: Proposed amended UNOS Policy 3.6. Briefing paper, February 1, 1–33. Richmond, VA: United Network for Organ Sharing.

———. 2002b. Proposals for public comment. August 21, 2002. Richmond, VA: United Network for Organ Sharing.

———. 2003. *2002 Annual report of the U.S. Scientific Registry of Transplant Recipients and the Organ Procurement and Transplant Network: Transplant data, 1992–2001.* Rockville, MD: U.S. Department of Health and Human Services.

———. 2006a. OPTN/UNOS Levies Member Sanction against St. Vincent Medical Center. Press release, March 2. Richmond, VA: United Network for Organ Sharing.

———. 2006b. OPTN/UNOS Declares Kaiser Permanente–San Francisco Medical Center a member not in good standing. Press release, December 13. Richmond, VA: United Network for Organ Sharing.

U.S. Department of Health and Human Services (HHS). 1989. A general notice of the health care financing administration. *Federal Register* 54 (1989): 51802–3.

———. 1994. Organ procurement and transplantation network. *Federal Register* 59 (1994): 46482–99.

———. 1996. Organ procurement and transportation [sic] network. *Federal Register* 61, no. 220 (1996): 58158–60.

———. 1998a. Organ procurement and transplantation network. *Federal Register* 63, no. 63 (1998): 16296–338.

———. 1998b. Medicare and Medicaid programs; hospital conditions of participation; identification of potential organ, tissue, and eye donors and transplant hospitals provision of transplant-related data. *Federal Register* 63, no. 119 (1998): 33856–75.

———. 1999. Organ procurement and transplantation network. *Federal Register* 64, no. 202 (1998): 56650–61.

———. 2000. Organ procurement and transplant network. *Federal Register* 65, no. 56 (2000): 15252.

———. 2006a. Response to solicitation on organ procurement and Transplantation Network (OPTN) living donor guidelines. *Federal Register* 71, no. 116 (2006): 34946–48.

———. 2006b. Spinal fusion for the treatment of low back pain secondary to degenerative disc disease. Meeting minutes of the Medicare Coverage Advisory Committee, Centers for Medicare and Medicaid Services, Baltimore.

———. 2007a. *American health information community successor.* White paper. August 6. Washington, DC: U.S. Goverment Printing Office.

———. 2007b. Medicare program: Hospital conditions of participation: Requirements for approval and re-approval of transplant centers to perform organ transplants. *Federal Register* 72, no. 61 (2007): 15197–280.

———. 2008. Medicare Part B physician/supplier national data, calendar year 2005 expenditures and service use by specialty (payment Amount). Washington, DC: Centers for Medicare & Medicaid Services. www.cms.hhs.gov/MedicareFeeforSvcPartsAB/Downloads/Specialty05.pdf.

U.S. General Accounting Office (GAO). 1993. *Organ transplants: Increased effort needed to boost supply and ensure equitable distribution of organs.* GAO/HRD-93–56. Washington, DC: U.S. Government Printing Office.

———. 1995. *Impact of organ allocation variances.* GAO/HEHS-95–203R. Washington, DC: U.S. Government Printing Office.

U.S. Government Accountability Office (GAO). 2004. *Medicare: CMS needs additional authority to adequately oversee patient safety in hospitals.* GAO-04–850. Washington, DC: U.S. Government Printing Office.

———. 2008. *Federal advisory committees: Issues related to independence and balance of advisory committees.* GAO-08–11T. Washington, DC: U.S. Government Printing Office.

U.S. Renal Data System (USRDS). 2007. *Annual data report: Atlas of chronic kidney disease and end-stage renal disease in the United States.* Bethesda, MD: National Institutes of Health. www.usrds.org/adr_2007.htm.

———. 2008. *Annual data report: Atlas of chronic kidney disease and end-stage renal disease in the United States.* Bethesda, MD: National Institutes of Health. www.usrds.org/adr_2008.htm.

Vermeule, Adrian. 2007. *Mechanisms of democracy: Institutional design writ small.* New York: Oxford University Press.

Vining, Aidan R., and Anthony E. Boardman. 1992. Ownership versus competition: Efficiency in public enterprise. *Public Choice* 32 (2): 205–39.

Vining, Aidan R., and Steven Globerman. 1998. Contracting out health care services: A conceptual framework. *Health Policy* 46 (2): 77–96.

Vining, Aidan R., and David L. Weimer. 1988. Information asymmetry favoring sellers: A policy framework. *Policy Sciences* 21 (4): 281–303.

———. 1990. Government supply and government production failure: A framework based on contestability. *Journal of Public Policy* 10 (1): 1–22.

———. 1997. Saintly supervision: Monitoring casino gambling in British Columbia. *Journal of Policy Analysis and Management* 16 (4): 615–20.

Wailoo, Allan, Jennifer Roberts, John Brazier, and Chris McCabe. 2004. Efficiency, equity, and NICE clinical guidelines. *British Medical Journal* 328 (7439): 536–37.

Walshe, Kiernan. 2003. *Regulating healthcare: A perspective for improvement.* Philadelphia: Open University Press.

Weber, Max. 1947. *The theory of social and economic organization.* New York: Oxford University Press.

Wehr, Elizabeth. 1984. System manipulated to get transplants for kids. *CQ Weekly* February 25:453–58.

Weaver, R. Kent. 1986. The politics of blame avoidance. *Journal of Public Policy* 6 (4): 371–98.

———. 1988. *Automatic government: The politics of indexation.* Washington, DC: Brookings Institution Press.

Weick, Karl E. 1984. Small wins: Redefining the scale of social problems. *American Psychologist* 39 (10): 40–49.

Weimer, David L. 1992. Claiming races, broiler contracts, heresthetics, and habits: Ten concepts for policy design. *Policy Sciences* 25 (2): 135–59.

———, ed. 1997. *The political economy of property rights: Institutional change and credibility in the reform of centrally planned economies.* New York: Cambridge University Press.

———. 2006. The puzzle of private rulemaking: Scientific expertise, flexibility, and blame avoidance in regulation. *Public Administration Review* 66 (4): 569–82.

Weimer, David L., and Aidan R. Vining. 2005. *Policy analysis: Concepts and practice,* 4th ed. Upper Saddle River, NJ: Pearson-Prentice Hall.

West, William. 2005. Administrative rulemaking: An old and emerging literature. *Public Administration Review* 65 (6): 665–68.

Weiss, Rick. 1996. Who should get liver transplants? *Washington Post,* December 9, A01.

Whitaker, Gordon P. 1980. Coproduction: Citizen participation in service delivery. *Public Administration Review* 40 (3): 240–46.

White, Joseph. 1999. Targets and systems of health care cost control. *Health Policy, Politics, and Law* 24 (4): 653–95.

Wilcox, Samantha A. 2003. Presumed consent organ donation in Pennsylvania: One small step for Pennsylvania, one great leap for organ donation. *Dickinson Law Review* 107 (4): 935–51.

Williamson, Oliver E. 1985. *The economic institutions of capitalism.* New York: Free Press.

Wilson, Robert. 1968. The theory of syndicates. *Econometrica* 36 (1): 119–52.

Wortman, Paul M., Amiram Vinokur, and Lee Sechrest. 1988. Do consensus conferences work? A process evaluation of the NIH Consensus Development Program. *Journal of Health Politics, Policy and Law* 13 (3): 469–98.

Yackee, Suan Webb. 2008. The hidden politics of regulation. Paper presented at the Annual Meetings of the Midwest Political Science Association, Chicago.

Yackee, Jason Webb, and Susan Webb Yackee. 2006. A bias toward business? Assessing interest group influence on the U.S. bureaucracy. *Journal of Politics* 68 (1): 128–39.

Young, Carlton J., and Robert S. Gaston. 2000. Renal transplantation in black Americans. *New England Journal of Medicine* 343 (21): 1545–52.

Zachary, Andrea A., John M. Hart, Stephen T. Bartlett, James Burdick, Paul Colombani, Lloyd E. Ratner, and Mary S. Laffell. 1997. Local impact of 1995 changes in the renal transplantation allocation system. *Transplantation* 63 (5): 669–74.

Ziliak, James P., David N. Figlio, Elizabeth E. Davis, and Laura S. Connolly. 2000. Accounting for the decline in AFDC caseloads: Welfare reform or the economy? *Journal of Human Resources* 35 (3): 570–86.

Index

195